ADMINISTRATION OF

COMPREHENSIVE NURSING CARE

ADMINISTRATION OF

Grace K. Eckelberry, R.N., B.S., M.N., M.S.

Associate Professor of Nursing
College of Nursing
University of Bridgeport
Bridgeport, Connecticut 06602

COMPREHENSIVE NURSING CARE

The Nature of Professional Practice

APPLETON-CENTURY-CROFTS
Educational Division
MEREDITH CORPORATION
New York

PRINTED IN THE UNITED STATES OF AMERICA
390-28693-1

Dedicated to my brother,
DR. NEIL E. ECKELBERRY,
whose courage and perseverance have inspired me.

Acknowledgments

Students, nurse-practioners, and faculty colleagues, all with a wide range of experience and educational background, have given the author insight into the vast potential for change in individual behavior and the inspiration to write the following chapters. Without them, the writer would have been unable to continue her efforts to define professional nursing practice. Miss Frances Reiter who has often expressed eloquently the scope of nursing care, has influenced significantly the author's comprehension of the nature of nursing care. Miss Reiter's reading of the first draft of the manuscript helped the author carefully weigh and evaluate what she had written.

The continuing encouragement of Mr. Charles Bollinger and the steadfast support of family members have made the labors of writing not only tolerable but often exciting. Finally, special acknowledgement must be given to Mrs. Ruth Newman, whose untiring attention to detail and meticulous work contributed to the preparation of the manuscript.

Preface

The last three decades have been marked by an amazing expansion of that unique and communicable body of knowledge which characterizes a profession and by an increasing demand for professional services. Some professions have been able to extend themselves by delegating technical functions to their assistants while retaining those functions which earmark the nature of that profession. Obviously, the success of such a delegation depends on the ability of a practicing group to define the nature and scope of the services it provides and to determine those services which require the professional practitioner. The extent to which nurses are able to accomplish these two tasks may have direct bearing on the issue: Is nursing a profession?

However, no one can deny that today many persons are involved in the act of giving nursing care. Wider participation has sharpened the differences in educational background, in previous experiences, in status, in job descriptions which include tasks to be performed. The result has often been a deplorable fragmentation of nursing care or a tremendous emphasis upon providing for, rather than giving, nursing care. Administration, the effective use of personnel and facilities to attain a goal, has become of paramount interest and importance as a process which helps to determine the quality of the product - in this case, the quality of nursing care.

Attempts to describe a desirable quality of nursing care have led to the use of such descriptive words as comprehensive, total, individualized, patient-centered, and family-centered. The compelling effort to determine the nature of nursing has resulted in a growing insistence that these qualitative terms be defined. What evidence is required, what indicators are used when nursing care is described as comprehensive, family-centered, or individualized?

The comprehensiveness of nursing care is determined by the comprehension of the one who gives or provides that care and the comprehension of the patient and family who receive it. Years of working with students in baccalaureate programs of nursing have made the writer well aware of the changes in the student's perception of nursing care. Simple concepts have become complex ones; the concept of nursing care as the giving of baths, treatments, and medications has changed to the concept of sustaining the patient's and family's defense mechanisms, and of reeducating the patient to another mode of life. Likewise, the years have shown changes in the patient's concept of nursing care. As the nurse has become a part of all phases of health and illness, patients perceive nursing care as giving emotional support, opening doors to resources, and helping to sort out reliable information.

Concepts form with the recognition that certain objects, phenomena, events, or behaviors have common characteristics. The characteristics may be as concrete as bathing, feeding, or toileting, or as abstract as supporting, rehabilitating, or counseling. As a concept becomes more abstract, it is increasingly necessary to study the process of concept formation itself.

The analysis of a process requires an understanding of the dynamics of change and the interaction of the elements in a situation. When the elements are human beings, the task of process analysis becomes more arduous but more challenging. Although the following chapters focus upon the nurse and her growing comprehension of the depth and scope of nursing care and its administration, it is always implied that the process of comprehending is affected deeply by the nurse's personal experiences with co-workers, patients and their families.

The following chapters are written for both nurse-practitioners and nurse-educators. The former may find suggestions that increase her comprehension of nursing care. She may be able to perceive the basic elements of administration in the act of giving direct care or in providing nursing care, whether she be staff nurse, team leader, clinical specialist, or administrator of nursing services. The nurse-educator may find some helpful ideas as to how to help the student through those difficult phases of assessment, planning, and evaluation in which she gives and provides for the nursing care of not one, but many patients and families in a variety of settings.

Perhaps both the reader and writer can move as does the chambered nautilus through a succession of more spacious chambers of their minds towards a greater comprehension of what nursing care involves and what then must be required of the professional nurse-practitioner.

Contents

The early chapters of this book are directed specifically to the nurse-educator. However, any reader will find here a description of that initial phase of growing self-awareness and attunement to another human being's frame of reference which is so essential to the self-realization of a nurse-practitioner.

Comprehension depends upon the personal frame of reference or the phenomenologic field in which differentiations are made and experiences are synthesized into meaningful wholes or systems of organizations. The kind of quality of the nursing care given is greatly determined by the comprehension of those who give it.

The author has chosen to describe how the nurse-educator who works with the beginning student may become aware of the latter's frame of reference. She may then select experiences which help the student change her perception of nursing and begin to relate purposefully to others. Continuous observation and sharing are emphasized.

A concept is defined as an arrangement or classification into categories of behaviors which have common characteristics. Concepts of health, illness, need, family, community, and problem-solving are described as significantly affecting the act of nursing.

ADMINISTRATION OF

COMPREHENSIVE NURSING CARE

PART I

The Nature of Comprehension: How It Is Changed

1

The Personal Frame of Reference

The Relationship between Comprehensive Nursing Care and the Comprehension of the Nurse

A growing concern with the improvement of the quality of nursing care has resulted in considerable effort to define kinds of nursing care. Some of the descriptive adjectives used have been technical, supportive, custodial, creative, comprehensive, and professional. Probably the adjective "comprehensive" has had the longest usage and enjoyed the greatest variety of interpretations. These have ranged from the care in which one nurse gives all the nursing care the patient needs during an assigned period of time to the nursing care which provides not only continuity but also extension of nursing care throughout the period the patient and his family require it.

The nurse-practitioner, the nurse-educator, the patient, the potential patient, and co-workers of the nurse have attempted to describe the components of comprehensive nursing care. In the last decade a committee of the National League for Nursing drafted a statement in which a patient was said to have a right to expect the following of modern nursing service:[1]

1. Nursing care necessary to help him regain or maintain his maximum degree of health.

2. Nursing personnel qualified through education, experience, and personality to carry out the services for which they are responsible.
3. Nursing personnel sensitive to his feelings and responsive to his needs.

When these descriptions and others are compared, certain common factors are apparent: the components of individualized care with the inclusion of family, the breadth and depth of the illness experience, the necessary problem-solving skills involving group planning and group evaluation. However, most striking is the ever present element of personal need to be matched by personal care given with deliberation and skill. In the final analysis, comprehensive nursing care is dependent upon the comprehension of those who provide that care. Comprehension is highly individual and changes with the individual as he makes use of his experiences, integrating them into more and more meaningful wholes, thereby increasing the breadth of his view and the depth of his understanding.

The Changing Phenomenologic Field

To change comprehension involves changing the personal frame of reference or the phenomenologic field described by Kurt Lewin, Donald Snygg, Arthur Combs, and others. Reality for the individual resides in his phenomenologic field which is made up of focus and margin, or figure and ground.[2] Snygg and Combs describe the first response of the individual as being a general response to the whole situation. Differentiation follows and depends upon the need of the individual or the use he can make of the components of his experience and upon the opportunities he has to make differentiations; for instance, time to make differentiations and enough like experiences to permit focuses to emerge in his field. What already exists in the phenomenologic field as differentiated determines to a large extent the future focus or foreground. For example, what the young student sees on the ward and describes as what nurses do depends greatly on how she has previously differentiated nursing in her own frame of reference from teaching, hostessing, social work, and so on.

The phenomenologic approach to individual behavior described by Snygg, Combs, and others places the *cause* of behavior entirely within the phenomenologic field or the personal frame of reference of the behaver. His action at any point of time is determined by the focuses or differentiations in his field at that time. Events and entities of common character which have been differentiated merge and become synthesized or integrated. It follows, then, that to change an individual's behavior it is necessary to bring about new differentiations within his field.

The Need for Wholeness

What causes the individual to differentiate, to select, and to bring into the foreground different entities and characters? The authors previously referred to cite the *need* of the individual to create and maintain some systems of organization which are uniquely his. This fundamental need determines the individual's phenomenologic field and, in turn, his behavior. Snygg and Combs describe this basic human need as the preservation and enhancement of the phenomenal self.[2] The self includes not only the physical, biologic organism but all things which the individual describes as "me." He seeks water, air, food, love, affection, social status, and prestige as an expression of his need to maintain an internal balance or wholeness. Physiologists have referred to this striving as the wisdom of the body, a systematic relevance or homeostasis.[2] Individual goals form because their achievement will satisfy a basic need of the individual. Methods of achieving the goals or techniques are developed.[2] Snygg and Combs distinguish techniques from habits, since the former require goals. Techniques persist because they have become differentiated by the individual as ways of achieving important goals.

From Ministration to Administration

How can the nurse-educator help the student nurse increase her comprehension of nursing care and develop the skills to administer it?

Often the learner brings with her a desire and a need to care for others. This motivation can be used to bring into the foreground of her phenomenologic field certain entities which, in turn, help her to enlarge her comprehension of nursing care. She observes, gives meaning to her observations, seeks more information, compiles this information, interprets and appraises her observations, setting a series of small goals. As she observes, she ministers or supervises those services which help the individual maintain and preserve his own defenses—bathing, toileting, feeding, resting, exercising, sheltering, positioning. These are the acts which nurture, nourish, sustain, and support the individual. A giving and receiving interaction and interchange occur between nurse and patient. The nurse's comprehension of the ill person and his immediate needs expands, and she sees him as a person with long-term health needs which must be met within the social setting of a family and a community.

As comprehension grows, direct ministration is supplemented by *ad*ministration in which the investigation and definition of nursing needs and the setting of long-term goals involve a group of individuals. No longer does this mean only the nurse and patient, but also the family, other nurses, and other members of the health team, such as the physician, the social worker, or the physical therapist. Organizing nursing care becomes more than reading an order, outlining an hourly work plan, assembling materials and equipment for a wound irrigation and dressing, communicating intelligibly with the patient, reporting and recording. Giving responsibility and delegating authority to others, coordinating activities, winning the cooperation of others, and evaluating the outcomes of action all are comprehended as components of nursing care.

The Developing Self-Concept

The nurse-educator, in accepting the personal theory of individual behavior, is able to determine the learner's frame of reference by observing her behavior. She has clearly in mind what changes in that frame of reference she desires to have take place. In other words, she has defined essential concepts and principles which the learner must use in giving the desired nursing care. She has developed methods or techniques to convey these concepts and principles to others.

Behavior is the response of the individual to his total environment, internal as well as external. Response includes thought, feeling, and action, and it may be overt—grossly observable, or covert—not demonstrated in action. Change in overt behavior means that reorganization in the phenomenal field has occurred and action has been taken to meet the behaver's need to preserve and enhance himself. In other words, he has established for the time being a balance or equilibrium with his total environment and has brought things into a harmonious relationship. He has learned. If the changes in behavior are desirable in terms of the educator's goals, then the educator can say he has taught.

As the nurse educator observes the learner's behavior, she draws upon her own background knowledge of the growth and developmental tasks of the individual. She perceives growth as progressive increase, a maturation process, one concerned with the achievement of size, stature, shape, and basic design. Development is the unfolding, the differentiation of sublayers, the refinement of shades and nuances which may be compared to flowering or blossoming. Development is greatly affected by the response to social environment and leads to self-concept and the image of self as others see one.

Perhaps more is known of growth tasks than of developmental tasks. However, certain developmental tasks have been well defined. For example, the tasks of becoming autonomous or independent, of becoming accepted as a member of a group (family or homologous or heterologous peer groups) have been outlined repeatedly. Other tasks are those of selecting a mate or a career, of becoming a parent, of working out a personal philosophy or system of beliefs. These tasks are carried out within a society with a particular culture or approved ways of behaving which that society has found most satisfactory for itself. Within the family, one of whose major functions is the transmission of culture, the individual learns what is acceptable behavior, what expectations are held for him. He incorporates in his own phenomenologic field what is meaningful to him, accepts for himself certain group goals, and works out techniques for meeting social as well as physical stresses. Patterns of adjustment are laid down and recognized by the individual as his self-knowledge increases. Always the preservation and enhancement of self is the basic need which may be expressed in *fight*, in *flight*, or in *conforming* behavior. Whatever the technique, the behavior is purposeful.

In the American culture, the developmental tasks of the youth and adult are somewhat sharply divided; the line is drawn somewhere in the early twenties. Youth is thought of as a period of exploration, of testing, of preparing for, or becoming. At some arbitrary point in time, at graduation from college or at attaining legal age, the youth becomes an adult overnight. He is classified and grouped. He now belongs to an economic, social, national, ethical, or ethnic class. He is expected not only to maintain a status but to advance it as well.

The individual approaches adulthood with images or reflections of occupational roles taken from the culture in which he lives. He may assimilate information from others who have seen and described nursing as bathing, feeding, toileting, carrying out the physician's orders, giving needles, relieving pain, and maintaining meals, supplies, and house-keeping. Whatever image the individual has of nursing, it creates expectancies with which he unconsciously compares and appraises what he later experiences, either as one who gives nursing care or one who receives it.

With the background knowledge just described of growth and developmental tasks, of the family and community culture from which students come, of society's images of nursing and nurses, the nurse-educator still needs to determine the meaning of the student's behavior as an expression of the student's phenomenologic field. Does the student's need to preserve and enhance her self-concept require that she protect, nurture, and nourish others, that she set things in order, or that she be in command or have authority to tell others what to do? Appraisal of the student's behavior as an expression of satisfaction of her needs is not easy. However, changes in the learner's frame of reference or phenomenologic field cannot be initiated by the nurse-educator without this appraisal. Acceptance of new concepts, awareness of the difference between one's own image of self and that held by others, cannot be expected until one determines what purposes the current behavior serves and what the behaver perceives as significant.

Summary

The kind of nursing care is greatly determined by the comprehension of those who give it. Comprehension depends upon the personal frame of reference or the phenomenologic field in which differentiations are made and experiences are synthesized into meaningful wholes or systems of organization. To preserve these systems means to preserve the self. All individual behavior has as its purpose the preservation and enhancement of the individual's self-concept. If behavior is to be changed, change must take place in the phenomenologic field.

The nurse-educator must strive to know the learner's personal frame of reference, to know what concepts are essential to giving comprehensive nursing care, and to find ways of placing these concepts within the grasp of the student. As they begin to appear within focus in the foreground of the student's field, changes in her behavior are inevitable, and the kind of nursing care given is modified.

References

1. National League for Nursing, Committee to Draft a Patient's Bill of Rights, What People Can Expect of Modern Nursing Service. Pamphlet.
2. Snygg, D., and Combs, A.W., Individual Behavior: A Perceptual Approach to Behavior, revised ed. New York, Harper & Brothers, 1959.

2

How the Personal Frame of Reference May Be Revealed

To change an individual's behavior, it is necessary to change his frame of reference and to bring about new differentiations within his phenomenologic field. The nurse-educator must determine what is the individual's present frame of reference. This chapter will present some ways in which the nurse-educator may gain insight into the learner's personal world. The beginning student will be presented as that learner, but the reader may also wish to substitute the senior student, staff nurse, patient, or family member in such a role.

A prerequisite to understanding another's personal frame of reference is some degree of self-insight, some awareness of one's own anxieties, hostilities, loneliness, and self-defenses which are ever in danger of threat. If she has achieved some measure of self-acceptance, the nurse-educator can feel with others more deeply, can enter more deeply into another's inner world, and help meet another's need to find new meanings and to reach out for self-fulfillment. The quality of compassion of which Arthur Jersild[1] writes is particularly essential in the nurse-educator, for her goal is to help students feel with others under the strain of illness, birth, and death—times when the self's defense systems have broken down, at least in part.

Perceptions Which the Beginning Student Brings to Nursing

For beginning students, small group experiences of faculty and students are selected because they not only stimulate interchange with peers but give the nurse-educator an approach to the student in that early period when the latter is less involved in the more complex nursing situation. The first expansion of comprehension may come when the student moves into a new residence situation, into a peer community where her associates come from widely different backgrounds.

A weekly three-hour group meeting of eight to ten students is suggested. The period is used to exchange ideas about nursing, individual health practices, kinds of illness experiences the student herself has had, her own reactions to other people in current living situations, the settings in which nursing occurs, information about her own community. The sharing of ideas and feelings about nursing may be stimulated by the small group discussing some or all of the following questions:

What word-picture do I have when someone says "nursing"?
What people have I seen doing nursing?
Where does nursing take place?
What does a nurse do?
Why do people choose to do nursing?
What kind of a person is a nurse?
How do people I know regard the work a nurse does?
How do the people I know regard nurses?
What does one get out of nursing?
What kinds of things should a nurse know?
How do people learn to nurse?

The student may be asked to answer some of the above questions individually in written form with the assurance that, should her answer or answers be used for discussion, her identity will be held in the strictest confidence.

The students could also be asked to bring to group discussion references to support or negate the following statements:

Nursing is valuable to the community.
Nursing is tedious, difficult, sometimes unpleasant.
Nurses are highly skilled.
Nurses tend to be bold, hard, and tough.

A reading list may be available with references which provide a brief look at how nursing was regarded in the past, how it is perceived today as a community service, and what some of the divergent views are as to what nursing and nurses mean to people.

The Significance of Previous Experiences

Since the major human experience in which the nurse becomes involved as a helping person is the illness experience, recalling some of her own illness experiences may help the student nurse bring into focus what was meaningful to her. With this awareness, she may be able to differentiate the components in the illness of another individual as she moves into nursing situations.

The student may be asked to write a description of one of her own illness experiences, being asked to try to "recapture" and set down her feelings about it. If she has none to recall, then she may describe the illness of a member of her immediate family. The description written only for the nurse-educator permits the student to share more freely than in a group. The emotional component of an illness experience is a major one, and to relate the experience may pose a threat to whatever strategies the individual self may have used to weave the experience into an idealized self; thus, some students may not share their emotional experiences. In any event, we know much is lacking in the reconstructed experience, since only what was useful to the self is remembered. Early in the development of self, the individual begins to identify with a group. Therefore, questions about family attitudes and interrelationships, if the individual in any way rejects or feels negatively about them, may be threatening to her; defenses are used to present to others what she would like her family to be.

Whatever individual accounts yield may be summarized objectively by the faculty leader and given to the group for discussion. This may help the student to become more aware of the common denominators in response to illness and to gain some insight into illness as a personal and family experience. In simple terms, some foundation can be given for the concepts of growth and development of personality in the family group. Students may be asked to keep the following questions in mind as they write of their illness experiences:

What changes took place in your plans?
What changes did your illness bring about within your family (e.g.,

reassignment of responsibilities, new responsibilities, changes in the family's daily schedule)?

What did you know about your diagnosis and what to expect?

How did you feel about being ill, about your diagnosis, about your recovery? Describe, if you can, how you expressed those feelings.

How did your family feel about your being ill? How did they show their feelings?

How did you feel about those people who cared for you—the physician, a parent, a sibling, another relative, a neighbor, a nurse, or others?

How has your family regarded the physician and/or nurse who attended the family during illness? For example, they may have regarded him or her as: one in authority who must be obeyed or impressed; a counselor to whom one tells any or all of his troubles; a stranger with whom one is not wholly comfortable; a person synonymous with trouble or calamity; a person associated with physical pain; a friend who cheers the family; a teacher who explains simply and clearly what has to be done; or a learned person who talks another language and is not understood.

What changes did this illness make in later health practices (e.g., choice of foods, sleep schedule, exercises and activities, etc.)?

What, if anything, did you and your family learn from this experience? Who helped you in your learning?

Do you feel these learnings could be acquired in other ways than by being ill?

Anxiety may be roused in the student when a faculty member invites her to talk about her family. The opposing or conflicting impulses and tendencies within every individual which have never been resolved but which she has succeeded in living with successfully may be brought into the foreground. The student becomes aware of what is and what she wishes would be; what is real and what is ideal. Very real anxiety results and may be expressed in many ways, often devious and obscure.[1] However, some students may be ready to share their experiences and therefore are willing, even relieved, to face their anxieties. Much depends upon the emotional relationship between student and faculty member. The exploration of personal family experiences may need to be initiated by the student, not the faculty member.

Arthur T. Jersild[1] writes of the inconsistency of impulses leading to inconsistent behavior which may be a revealing clue to anxiety. The impulse to evade anxiety may lead to resistance in various forms. Flight reactions may be expressed by flight into words, by treating emotional problems as though they were logical problems, by avoiding any intimate emotional relationship, or by diluting the personal meaning of what is threatening by discoursing on impersonal aspects. Work may be resorted to as an endeavor to blunt or avoid anxiety.

Similarities and differences in family groups may be given to the group in a summary made by the faculty member, or she may use a family study as a springboard for group discussions. The family study frequently initiates sharing of personal experiences, and the student may feel more secure initially, discussing another family than her own. Some helpful information can be evoked by the questions listed below, but it is to be held in strictest confidence by the faculty member.

Who are the members of your family; what is their relation to each other as to age?

What goals are common to all the members of your family?

What things does your family do best together?

Which of your needs does your family meet most successfully? Least successfully? Not at all?

Do you expect specific and different things from each member of your family? What are the roles or parts they always seem to take?

What part do you see yourself playing in your family group?

What events have occurred within your family group which have caused crises? Why did these events cause crises?

How does your family regard food? What attitudes or habits do they have about the selection, preparation, and serving of foods? How do you feel about mealtime in your family?

How does your family regard rest and sleep? What, if any, practices are accepted as family habit?

How does your family regard play and recreation? What plans are made for it as part of the family's daily schedule? Is vacation time planned as a family affair?

How does your family regard health? (Check those statements that are appropriate, and add others.)

Health is a privilege one earns through the daily observance of certain practices of balanced living.

Health is present when there are no physical complaints. Health is present when it is not necessary to receive medical attention.

Health is guaranteed by periodic physical examinations and pre-scribed immunizations.

Health is affected by spiritual and emotional as well as physical needs. Emotional disturbances can create physical symptoms.

The degree of well-being can be measured by one's zest for living and working.

Physical symptoms always involve emotions.

A group discussion of cultural patterns within the family group that affect health and illness may be initiated by the faculty member's use of a family study. Food, of course, always provides a fascinating subject when it is approached as a symbolic language and a means of relating one's self to others. The discussion of observance of holidays within the home, of anniversaries and other events which involve the family group, may lead to a discussion of more intimate levels of family life such as birth, death, weddings, christenings, coming of age, and so on. This lays the foundation upon which a concept of culture may be built.

Self-awareness

To what extent is the student conscious of her reactions to others and of the reactions she evokes in others? Sharing this self-awareness with the faculty member at a time when her interpersonal relationships are in no way regarded as therapeutic may help her develop some beginning understanding of the use of self. The *"therapeutic* use of self" may then become meaningful at a later date.[2] The following questions may be provocative:

How do I feel about my roommate?
What have been my difficulties in adjusting to a roommate, housemates, faculty members?
What groups am I acquainted with who differ greatly from my own group in regard to religion, housing, customs, food?
What prejudices do I know I have?
How do I behave when I am with someone whom I respect? With someone whom I dislike?
How do I behave when someone disagrees with me or ignores me?
How do I behave when someone gives me orders to be carried out?
How do I think my teachers feel about me?
What kinds of things do my friends select to do when they invite me to spend time with them?
What kinds of things do my friends choose to confide in me?
What actions on my part have caused people to withdraw from me? To ignore me? To oppose me? To resent me? To defy me?
In what ways have I been able to attract people to me, to win their confidence?

In order to know something of the student's awareness of other groups than her family and her perception of nursing as a community service, group discussion can begin with the following questions:

What is the name of your community? What is its size in square miles and in population numbers?
What do you know of its origin and history?
What do you know of the groups within it—ethnic and cultural groups, economic groups, work groups, religious groups, professional groups, and so on?
What are the educational resources in your community? To what extent are they used?
What do you see to be the needs of the citizens in your community? Which ones are met through organized community agencies and how? Which ones have not been met, and why, in your opinion, is this so?
How do you see yourself as a nurse working in your own community? What do you think a nurse might do to help meet community needs?

Experiences Which Increase Comprehension

In addition to small group discussions, observation-participation experiences may be arranged in settings where nursing care is being given—e.g. in the hospital ward, home, industry, or nursing home. Group or individual interviews with resource people may be arranged as the student's growing interests lead her to seek more information. Films are sometimes used to provide a vicarious experience in a setting too complex for observation-participation such as the clinic or school.

Individual conferences with the faculty group leader should occur frequently. To make these possible in a busy class schedule, periods set aside for the small group experiences may be used by some group members for library study and independent reading, and individual conferences are held at scheduled times.

In short, exploration of the student's phenomenologic field is accompanied by experiences not only appropriate to her current interests but sufficiently provocative to open for her new vistas and new avenues to travel. The amount of participation increases as the student becomes comfortable in new situations and makes use of the knowledge and skills she already possesses. It is at this point that specific nursing techniques are introduced. Techniques are selected which, when skillfully used, aid and support the adaptive mechanisms of the ill person. The techniques chosen are related to: providing rest, controlled activity, and diversion; permitting free communication of fears, anxieties, confusion, and hostility; maintaining adequate nutrition; and controlling physical environment. Sustaining or supportive nursing care is emphasized. Therapeutic and reeducative nursing care, since it requires specific information from curative and rehabilitative medical care, is regarded as more advanced and is reserved until the student is ready to help the more dependent patient.

Observation-participation experiences in nursing situations often provide even more insight as to how the student perceives nursing, and as to what are her own expectations of a nurse and nursing. Arrangements may be made for the new student to accompany an older student or staff nurse as she works with a patient. Careful selection must be made of a nurse whose attention and concern is with the patient, rather than the tasks she is performing. The student must be carefully oriented to observe what the patient says, does, how he looks, his posture and gestures, his response to what the nurse says and does. Some briefing as to the kinds of things the nurse does to show her concern for the patient and to make him comfortable will help the student observer participate to some degree and therefore feel more at ease. Arranging pillows, giving foot-room in upper bed coverings, tightening or slipping a draw-sheet, positioning a patient in bed, preparing him for meals, serving trays, feeding the patient who needs help—these and many other small acts may be reviewed, observed, and performed jointly. Students will vary greatly as to what first impresses them. Some are preoccupied with what the nurse does. Others very quickly have much to report of what they heard, saw, and felt. Great emphasis is placed on looking and *listening.* Care must be taken that judgment of the meaning of behavior is not encouraged. Rather, the approach is: What was I feeling and thinking; what more could I look for; what was the stimulus or stimuli that produced the response I observed?

Free narrative writing in a kind of diary form can provide a record of a continuing experience between the patient and nurse. Some nurse-educators have used tape recordings made immediately after the experience as an unstructured process to record continuing experiences with a patient. The student often becomes aware of her own developing skills in observation, and exhibits increasing curiosity as to the causes of interaction. When students share their written observations of the same situation with each other, they become aware of differences in perception and in what is real to the individual.

The nurse-educator finds innumerable opportunities to introduce content on means of communication, the techniques of asking open-ended questions, and the choice of words. Whatever knowledge content on interviewing is introduced, it is done when the student shows that she is ready to make use of it.

Using the same guide, the nurse-educator introduces definite nursing procedures related to sustaining and supporting the patient's own defenses. For example, nursing measures which help preserve the defenses of the skin, mucous membranes, postural balance, cell nutrition, and elimination of waste, if taught concurrently with simple techniques related to the orientation of and communication with the patient, help the student become increasingly aware of the whole self.

The observation-participation experiences in nursing situations reveal much of the individual student. Her response to and use of these experiences give many clues to her frame of reference, her prevailing patterns of behavior, and the differentiations she begins to make. The anecdotal record is an excellent tool to help the nurse-educator form a portrait of the student, assess specific learning needs, and select individual learning experiences.

Visits with a nurse to other community settings may be used to help the student associate nursing with people wherever they may be, to see illness as beginning and ending in the home and community, and to relate nursing to health and well people, as well as to sickness and the ill. Such visits need to be carefully planned with orientation of those who are visited, as well as the student-visitor. In no way are the experiences intended to introduce the students to the many fields of nursing or to give her knowledge of an organized community agency. She is simply given the opportunity to enlarge her view of nursing as part of meeting people's health needs wherever and whenever they occur and to expand her view of the nurse as a person who responds and relates to people.

Summary

The beginning experiences described in this chapter provide a way in which the nurse-educator and the student can share and grow together. Not only have ways to discover another's world been described, but ways to effect change in the phenomenologic field of the beginning student have been introduced. If the nurse-educator believes that the act of becoming a nurse requires finding new meanings and a change in one's self, she covets any experience for the student which may be significant to her and involves her as a whole person. The nurse-educator never loses sight of the fact that she, too, is involved in and is a part of the learning experience. She often needs to examine her own beliefs, values, and attitudes, since they play a vital part in changing the student's inner world.

References

1. Jersild, A.T. When Teachers Face Themselves. New York, Bureau of Publications, Teachers College, Columbia University. 1955.
2. Peplau, H. Inter-Personal Relations in Nursing: A Conceptual Frame of Reference for Psycho-Dynamic Nursing. New York, G.P. Putnam's Sons. 1952.

3

Concepts Which Extend One's Comprehension of Nursing Care

When some of the similarities in the many definitions of comprehensive nursing care are recognized, it is possible to identify basic concepts which need to be differentiated and accepted by the student. A concept may be thought of as a category of phenomena, events, or behaviors, which have common characteristics.[1] A concept may be a very simple, concrete one such as the concept of a chair, a box, a cat. On the other hand, it may be abstract and very complex, encompassing many subconcepts. The concept of intelligence is abstract and complex; memory is a subconcept of intelligence. Immunity, an extremely complex concept, has within it the subconcepts of antigen, the agent, the anamnestic response, and so on.

Concepts grow out of observation of single instances, from direct or vicarious experiences. The child observes fur, tail, four feet, whiskers, a meow and a purr, hears the term "cat," sees the picture labeled cat, and begins to classify an animal with these common characteristics as a cat. Instances of behavior with certain common characteristics and described as courageous leads the individual to build the concept of courage, an abstraction based on a cluster or constellation of ideas with commonalties which help him to classify a behavior under one heading. Man as a thinking being must work with concepts in order to place or arrange his experiences in some kind of order. The shifting, sorting, and rearrangement that takes place in the phenomenologic field results in conceptualization which preserves the wholeness or integrity of the self.

The nurse-educator whose goal is to increase the individual's comprehension of nursing care must have certain basic concepts well described in order to be able to help the student change her frame of reference. This chapter attempts to describe the concepts of health, illness, the family and community as related to health and illness, and the concept of problem-solving.

Health

Nursing is concerned with restoring people to health, helping them maintain and promote health. In many settings nursing is predominantly concerned with the promotion of health, which implies degrees or variances in the individual's state of health. The "well" person may become "more well." For many years, nursing used the term "positive health," but this phrase has now been discarded. It was used to help develop the concept of health as a state of being in which the *individual* was able to contribute *his* most and to live what *for him* was an abundant life. In other words, the human being in his constant effort to maintain stability with his internal and external environment has points at which he can make best use of himself in the situations in which he moves. He not only *gives* his best but *is* his best; not only *does,* but *is*; realizes himself as well as produces.

Health is highly individual, a nonstatic and dynamic concept. To help the individual restore, maintain, or promote his health is to understand what requirements for optimum being and giving are not being met and which of these must be supplied. When a requirement is not met, a need exists. Thus, the concept of need may be considered a subconcept of health; the initial step is to identify needs or unmet requirements. Which requirements can be met by the individual himself? What needs does he perceive to be lacking, and what resources does he have to fulfill them? Until he becomes aware of these deficiencies and accepts the initiative for fulfilling them, he remains dependent and is not stabilized. Health requirements must be supplied for him.

Because he is a biosocial being, his requirements may be predominantly biologic, psychosocial or spiritual, but all these requirements are necessary for health. With this interpretation, it is easily apparent why health has sometimes been made synonymous with wholeness, with the integration of self or being which makes the life abundant possible.

Illness as a State of "Dis-ease"

When the individual is no longer at ease, no longer in relative comfort with his total environment, he experiences dis-ease which, at varying degrees, is recognized as illness by himself and by others. He may simply feel ill at ease (malaise), vaguely uncomfortable, or acutely distressed. Dysfunction may progress to actual irreversible organic change. When dis-ease is sufficiently localized in tissues, organs, or in a behavior pattern, a disease entity can be described in terms of etiology, a constellation of signs and symptoms, onset, course, and sequelae. The stages of disease are often delineated as prodromal, acute, chronic, and convalescent. When these terms are applied to dis-ease, they depict the arc of imbalance through which the individual may move toward or away from stability or equilibrium within his own world and with his environment.

Illness has meaning or significance to the individual within his own frame of reference or phenomenologic field. Certain common determinants affect the meaning of illness to the individual, such as the kinds of physiologic imbalances present, the foreground of his field and the pressures of the sociocultural situation in which he lives. However, illness is a unique experience for every individual and will be used in a way peculiar to him.

As a human being, the individual is at any point in his life span engaged in developmental tasks, tasks which relate his self to others. Dis-ease, the illness experience, is superimposed upon an ongoing developmental sequence and will have different meanings or degrees of significance to the individual at different points in his development. This is clearly recognized when the child becomes ill and his task of becoming autonomous or of being accepted by his peer group is interrupted. Unfortunately, less recognition is given to the impact of illness upon the adult's task of holding a job, of maintaining a position, or of relating himself to the universe.

Biologically, the individual has certain compensating mechanisms which come into play in states of dis-ease; for example, dilation and

constriction of the peripheral vascular system, hyper- and hyposecre-
tion of hormones, hyper- and hypoventilation of the respiratory
system, shifts in fluid and electrolyte balance. Other mechanisms or
patterns are developed as modes of defending and enhancing the self or
ego.

Stanley H. King writes of the *ego adaptive* mechanisms which are
conscious and flexible.[2] Examples of these are avoidance, transference,
and sublimation. More rigid unconscious and repetitive patterns are
called *ego defense* mechanisms. Examples of these are repression,
projection, denial, and reaction formation. Dorothy Crowley describes
defense mechanisms as "basically symbolic self-deceptions which the
ego uses to ward off situations which provoke anxiety and other
disturbing emotions."[3] She refers to the basic structure of patterns of
response to stressful situations which are laid down in childhood and
which are used again and again because they have proved effective.
Thus, fight, flight, withdrawal, or passive behavior become highly
characteristic of the way the individual has selected to preserve his
integrity, his wholeness of self.

King describes a third group of mechanisms as the *ordering*
mechanisms.[2] These serve "to provide continuity from one situation to
the next" and "to give a structure to one's psychological world." They
are the woof which binds together the warp of daily experience. King
cites beliefs, attitudes, and values as ordering mechanisms. He states:

Beliefs include knowledge, opinions, and faith about aspects of the
world; they are the pattern and meaning of a thing. In their clear state
beliefs are emotionally neutral." . . . Attitudes are in part a readiness to
act; in addition to cognitive properties there are affective or emotional
qualities which we often call "pro" or "anti." Values are principles by
which we establish priorities and hierarchies of importance among
needs, demands, and goals, helping us to decide where our emotional
investments will be made and the extent of these investments.

Beliefs, attitudes, and values affect the individual's perception of
illness and shape its meaning for him. If he believes pain is the penalty
for misdoing, if he is ready to resentfully reject an authority figure, if
he values his own goals to the exclusion of his family's—then he may
perceive illness as retribution, those who care for him as jailors, and his
plans for the future as unalterable. Illness will have a very different

meaning for the individual who regards pain as a protective device or a warning to seek help, who tends to trust authority as evidence of expertise, and who relates his own goals to those of the group with whom he is immediately closely associated.

The Family as the First Group Experience

Within the family the personality is developed and culture is transmitted. This is the individual's first "other world," and within it the early developmental tasks are begun. Here the individual begins to distinguish himself from others, to experience trust, to receive love, to be accepted, to accept others, and to develop an image of the self which others see. Here he learns ways of acting, thinking, and feeling which have been tested by the group and found successful over past generations.[4] These learned ways of the past serve as a design for living and determine to a large degree how he perceives his environment and how he differentiates, selects, and integrates his experiences into his personal frame of reference. The family comprises the individual's first group experience. This is his first experience with a group entity with definite membership, with common goals and a feeling of belonging-ness, with definite positions and roles described for and accepted by its members.

Like the individual, the family has stresses from outside and from within and strives for a measure of balance or coordinated control to prevent it from being overwhelmed by the barrage of stimuli in excess of its capacity to accomodate. Religious, moral, social, racial, and economic forces, the pressure of mores and customs are some of the stresses from without; from within, basic biologic bonds of man and woman as mates, parent and child, serve as centripetal or centrifugal forces. As with the individual, functional integrity is achieved by the processes of identification, differentiation, focus, motivation, and integration.[5-6]

No family is wholly adequate or wholly stable. However, some criteria can be used to estimate its measure of adequacy. Do the members know and accept their individual roles? Are members willing to accept group goals? Does the family group attempt to provide for the physical and emotional needs of the members? Is it possible to give security and affection to each other? Are the parents able to select what is useful from their individual cultural backgrounds so that understanding between parents, and parents and children, is possible? In other words, are cultural conflicts resolved?

Earl Lomon Koos describes cycles in the life of a family with developmental tasks which must be performed.[7] In the adjustment stage, a permanent sexual role as well as the roles of husband and wife must be developed. The position of a married couple is attained and accepted. Child-bearing brings new roles with a change in attitudes and values. Physical as well as financial responsibilities undergo a shift. During the child-rearing stage, the parental role is accepted, and the needs of the child must be made compatible with personal and marital needs. As the family group expands, the incorporation of new members places many strains upon the group.

As the child is launched, the family group undergoes the weaning experience, the task of giving emotional independence to the adolescent member and helping him prepare for his responsibilities to society. The family group contracts only to be extended as the new roles of in-law and grandparent are developed, and husband and wife roles are resumed to a fuller extent. The loss of a mate, with its impact upon the family group, also creates new adjustments.

The family as a group has the dual task of attaining its goals and meeting the needs of its individual members. With increased knowledge of group process, recognition has been given to the importance of this dual task if the group is to remain a true group—that is, if it is to preserve its wholeness with members accepting and playing their individual roles, and if it makes possible the development of individual personalities. At times one task assumes priority but the complete exclusion of either has a disintegrative effect upon the family group.

The stability of the family is a delicate thing made up of the interplay and exchange between members. Crises occur when a change in role is necessary and the emotional balance within the family group is disturbed. Illness of an individual member often creates a difficult change in role and a crisis occurs. As with the individual, the stage of development at which illness is interjected affects the nature and severity of the crisis for the family. A family crisis may serve to bring about greater solidarity or to dissolve the boundaries which make the family a whole.

Within the family group the individual formulates his perception of health, illness, birth, and death. He learns to view his body as good or shameful, to express his emotions in ways acceptable to the group, to perceive pain as punishment or as a signal for action. Certain symptoms he learns to view as meriting help outside the family; others are always treated by self-medication. Birth may be regarded as an illness with attendant isolation and great anxiety, or as a natural event of great significance—a family event warranting the gathering of relatives and the use of many symbols to signify its importance.

In some cultures, sleep is thought of as "a little death;" therefore, sleep is often resisted in illness. No one in the family ever sleeps alone in a room, and often all the male children sleep in one room and all the female in another. Death may be made bearable by many rituals and a period of mourning in which grief may be given full expression. As at birth, the family gather, often remaining together for a period of time. In some other cultures, as at times in our own, the subject of death is shunned and avoided, and the child is protected from any contact with it. It is not uncommon to find the young American adult has never viewed the dead, never attended a funeral, and is unfamiliar with the rituals of burial.

When the body is regarded as housing the man, a residence to be kept in good repair, the so-called "intrusive procedures" necessary in illness may be acceptable. On the other hand, if the body is regarded as inviolate, operative procedures are thought to desecrate the temple of the body, and autopsies are never performed.

One of the cultural values transmitted by the family is that of the relationship of man to other men. Stanley H. King,[2] quoting Florence Kluckholn, describes the possible relationship as lineal, collateral, or individualistic. The lineal relationship stresses the continuity of groups through time. This cultural value holds dear the long line through generations of group goals. The goals of the "laterally extended group" at a given point of time is described as the collateral relationship of man to men, while the individualistic relationship gives primacy to individual goals rather than group goals. Whatever the cultural value, it is of great significance in shaping the individual's perception of illness and in determining the family's illness experience. Some families accept and take an active part in the illness of a member in another generation, while others are only involved in the illness of a member of the immediate group. In still other families, the illness concerns only the individual member, and his action is determined by his own goals and directions.

One of the areas in family living in which cultural factors are most apparent is that of food patterns. The first emotional experience of the individual is associated with food. With food comes warmth and security; with new foods, their flavors, textures, and colors may be associated with fear, tension, and anxiety. Food begins to speak a language; it is a mode of communication between the individual and the group in which he has his first social role. Food also relates the individual to the past. It has been said that the story of food is the historical progression of man's struggle for survival. During the course of this struggle, man has selected certain food symbols to represent his relationship to nature and to supernatural forces. Certain foods are associated with religious beliefs: for example, the bitter and the sweet foods used by the Jew; the wafer shared with the family and guests at Christmastime in the Polish family; and the 21 items, each with its own meaning, so carefully prepared for the Christmas feast. The special cakes of all varieties used in many cultures for births, baptisms, weddings, or funerals were originally sacrificial offerings.

Food symbols abound in folklore. The planting and harvesting of the grain seeds from which the staff of life is produced, be it rice, wheat, oats, barley, or rye, have always been occasions for singing, dancing, and storytelling. Crusts of bread in the baby's cradle bestow upon him creative power. Milk and honey are symbols of abundance. Eggs symbolize fertility. Potatoes are endowed with healing power. The apple is associated with perpetual youth, the orange with the virtues of chastity and eternal love, while the plum and peach bespeak longevity and immortality.

The individual family selects from its cultural heritage those customs and folkways related to food which have significance for the group. The parents' own family experiences with foods which gave each of them comfort, security, and the warm glow of companionship and affection, affect greatly the food patterns developed within the immediate family. Food preferences are also related to who prepared and provided the food, to the utensils and dishes used in preparing the food, to the area in the home where food was prepared and served, to the foods served when a family member became ill, or to the foods for which the town or region is noted (New England baked beans, Southern grits and hominy, Wisconsin cheese).

Within a complex culture there are subcultures. A regional, urban, rural, religious, or minority group affiliation will create significant differences.[4] A family has its own individual cultural pattern, having selected and preserved from its cultural heritage what is meaningful to it. Its pattern will have certain likenesses to other families of similar affiliation so that the family will feel comfortable and at ease within the groups in which it moves. From the family, then, as it moves through its life cycle carrying out its development tasks and selecting its own cultural forms, emerge the individual's perceptions of health and illness, his beliefs, values, and attitudes.

The Community

The community is often described sociologically as the smallest social unit that can maintain and support itself. Communication is the essential factor in the development of a community. People drawn together by a common bond of physical proximity and interaction form a neighborhood which is able to sustain itself and to supply its needs for foodstuffs, money exchange, schools, places of worship, recreation, and social exchange. In folk society, communication is by word of mouth, face-to-face contact. As neighborhoods grow in size and coalesce, communication depends upon secondary or mass media, such as the newspaper, radio, and television. Towns and cities emerge, ranging from the metropolis to the megalopolis.

The growth of communities within a community is observable today in the phases of community development such as centralization, concentration, segregation, invasion, succession, and decentralization. The initial centralization may have resulted from the need of traders to exchange their goods and from the demands for cargo to be transported by rail or waterway. Families began to cluster about these fixed points, and services needed by all began to concentrate in some central area.

Residence and shop or marketplace then became discrete or separate. Expansion resulted in invasion of residence areas, and the succession of homes replaced by stores and offices began. Eventually, distance and the formation of new neighborhoods led to decentralization, so that today the phrases "the greater city area" (versus the city proper), "exurbia," and "rurban" have replaced the earlier distinction between city and suburb. The core of the original city often consists of stores, banks, markets, and offices, the only residents being people who have not been able to move away because of economic reasons or lack of motivation. Wealth and leadership are often located in the outer city, while the preponderance of social, health, and economic needs are found in the core city. Suburban residents' resistance to assuming responsibility for those who reside in the inner city and the urban residents' resentment of that rejection result in tremendous community conflict.

A community has certain characteristics which affect its health needs. The diagnosis of its health needs and the defining of its health problems may be approached in much the same way one determines those factors which predispose an individual to illness and disease. What information is needed? What information is available and where or how may it be found? Data concerning the following can be of assistance:

1. The size of the population; the trend and rate in population growth. (Is it expanding or decreasing, rapidly or slowly?)
2. The kind of population change. Are laborers and semiskilled workers moving into a quiet village? Is the influx of population from another region, race, or culture? Is it predominantly an older or younger group?
3. The age and sex distribution of the population.
4. The general vitality of the population. What are the specific mortality rates; morbidity rates; prevalence and incidence rates of specific diseases?
5. The socioeconomic-cultural configuration of the population. What is the average family income? How many women are working; of what age; at what kind of work? What is the average level of formal schooling? What kind of housing? Is it a striving community with social classes changing rapidly?
6. Physical environmental factors such as sources of food and water supply, playground space, provisions for disposal of human and other waste, topography.
7. Organized efforts of the community to govern itself, to meet its health and social needs. What agencies, health and social, have been created either through legislation or voluntary action?

8. Patterns of medical care. Is medical care from private physicians, clinics, or the medical specialist? Where are babies born? Is the midwife used; what is her preparation or that of her alternate? What is the average hospital stay? What other institutions are used for care of the ill?

A community has a structure, both formal and informal. Its formal structure is found in its institutions concerned with government, industry, health, religion, and education—in other words, in its town council, its governmental offices, its schools and churches, it departments of health and labor, its organizations of industrial management and finances. Within this formal structure may be found what are sometimes called the dominant groups of the community. In these groups reside the resources of money, legal provisions, administrative and professional leadership. Final decisions are made within the dominant groups.

On the other hand, sub-dominant groups make up the informal structure of a community. The subdominant groups may be made up of laborers, housewives, semiprofessionals and professionals. These groups have access to and express the community's feelings. They wield significant influence in a community and affect greatly the decisions made by the dominant groups. The check exerted by subdominant groups is often discernible in the inertia and sometimes frank resistance of a community to the recommendations of professionally conducted community surveys, or in the failure of a legislative act to bring about reform. It is the wise community health worker who studies carefully and systematically the power systems of his community. Who are the "right" people, the people who exercise influence, who initiate movement? The right people in one orbit of community action may not be the right people in another. Community action often results from the timed interaction of the forces which exist in an event, in people, and in the organizations with which they associate themselves.[8]

A community agency is a means or instrument empowered by the people to carry out group decisions. It has its origin in group concern and group planning. Community agencies may be classified with respect to the community needs with which they deal—for example, health, social, or group work agencies. Another classification finds its basis in the source of financial support or the group by whom the agency has been empowered—for example, official, voluntary, or professional agencies. Nursing service takes place within the framework of a community agency. The scope of that service is affected by the nature of the agency and by the group goals which the agency has been empowered to achieve.

Problem-Solving

If the nurse-educator perceives comprehensive nursing care as including the diagnosis of nursing problems, the selection of immediate and long-term goals, the institution of a plan of nursing care, and its evaluation leading to possible revision and further nursing diagnosis, then the concept of problem-solving is an integrated part of her frame of reference.

Before describing the process of problem solving, one must look at the nature of a problem. A situation which requires an answer to a question in the absence of reliable information concerning the appropriate procedure to be adopted, occurs because a problem exists.[9] The problem exists because the individual feels some obstacle blocks the attainment of a goal or objective. How to remove that obstacle is the problem and the individual becomes aware of the problem after he feels the presence of the obstacle.[10] The feeling or concern must exist before the problem can be recognized and is the initial phase of the problem-solving process. John Dewey in *How We Think*[11] called this feeling a "felt difficulty." Such a feeling is basic to the recognition of the obstacle to be removed or the definition of the problem. What takes place, then, in problem solving? What is the process?

Much goes on between the feeling and the formulation of the question to be answered or the definition of the problem. The situation is surveyed, some reconnoitering is done, and factors in the situation are investigated. Then the question to be answered is selected. Already a certain amount of weeding has been done; some of the factors in the total situation have been eliminated. Once the problem has clearly emerged, the process of problem solving continues with the search for possible answers or tentative solutions. These may be thought of as guesses, hunches, "suppose we do this," or a possible hypothesis stated as related cause and effect.

All possible solutions are tested by reasoning out possible consequences. Some are eliminated because it is found they have been tried by others and found wanting. Some are not compatible with basic assumptions or deductions already made by the individual (those things he now takes for granted). The most reasonable solution or solutions are selected to be tested in the actual situation. If not wholly successful, the solution is refined or discarded and other solutions considered.

The problem-solving process as with all processes, is dynamic and not always sequential. As possible answers to the question are sifted through the reasoning which relates cause and effect, other factors in the situation often emerge and the problem is redefined.

In summary, the individual who becomes engaged in problem solving has a goal which has grown out of an interest or a concern which mobilizes him to attain some end. He feels a difficulty, some impediment to reaching that goal and becomes aware of an obstacle. Inquiry leads to identifying the obstacle. This is investigated, and a question to be answered emerges. Possible answers or actions which may serve to remove the obstacle are posed and thought through in terms of consequences. These may be ascertained by seeing if that answer or action has ever been applied by others, or the probable consequences may be screened through the assumptions which have grown out of the individual's previous experiences. The most relevant answer or answers are put to test in the real situation, the results evaluated and the answer revised, discarded, or further elaborated.

The following situation may illustrate the process of problem solving:

Marie Tyler, a staff nurse serving as team leader, has become much interested in the follow-up care of patients. With the hospital stay for the individual patient becoming more and more brief, she is aware that the discharged patient frequently goes home with medical or nursing care or both still needed. She has concentrated in team conferences on teaching patients as much self-care as possible. However, discharge orders are frequently written on the day of discharge so that any orderly, progressive teaching plan is impossible. She discusses the ward situation with her team and with the head nurse. All agree that plans for discharge are never shared, probably because physicians are not aware of the preparation needed by the family and the patient to shift his care from hospital to home. The physician has a detailed medical care plan and carefully evaluates the response of the patient to that plan, but therapy includes more than this. The problem seems to be: How can those needs of the patient which will require extension of health care be recognized early by the professional health team who work with him on Ward X in Hospital Y?

Possible answers were posed by members of the nursing team and the head nurse. Perhaps a planned conference with family members at the time of admission would reveal factors in the home situation which would predict the need for extended care by professional health workers or the use of other resources than the family's. Another suggestion proposed an early planned interview with the patient concerning his work and home situation. One team member was convinced that teaching all patients self-care when possible, or routinely teaching some family member any nursing procedure which can be carried out in the home, would eliminate the problem. One nurse who was well-known for her keen observations of patient's behavior suggested that the head nurse select those patients whose clinical charts present factors which may persist and perpetuate the illness, and that biweekly conferences be arranged to share observations and to interpret them in terms of continuing health needs. The resident or a member of the medical staff, the nurse(s) caring for the patients selected, the medical social worker on the hospital service, and a public health nurse (alternately appointed for three months by the local voluntary public health nursing agency and the city health department) would be constant members of this conference group.

Which answer was the most probable solution to the problem? Each was thoroughly discussed with some exploration of what had happened when a particular solution had been applied in other situations either known to the team members and head nurse or actually tried out by them in other hospitals.

Often an adult member is admitted without a family member present. However, if he or she is present, not always does that member play the key role in the family group. Early in his hospital stay, the patient is not able to select from his home and work situation the factors which best reveal the need for extended care. The teaching of self-care and nursing procedures assumes that the need for continued ministration to physical needs is the only cause for extending care. What of the patient who needs to accept a dietary regime and to carry it out, to understand better what signs and symptoms must be reported to a physician, to work out a rest and activity regime as the homemaker in a busy household? Is not the best solution the pooling of the observations of key members of the health team who see the patient frequently, who relate to him differently, and who know the immediate community and may even know the family from which the patient comes.

The tentative solution selected was the bi-weekly conferences centering around patients selected by the head nurse. The conferences proved most productive in identifying needs for extension of care as evidenced by the patient's behavior. The medical social worker was most helpful in suggesting ways to improve communication with patients but felt she could be on call for those conferences in which she either knew the patient or the socioeconomic needs of the patient were in question. Likewise, the public health nurse felt a weekly attendance at the conference would make her knowledge of the community available to the conference group with possible exploration of other ways to share general information.

It would seem that Marie Tyler moved through the problem-solving process which began with her feeling that the restoration of patients to their fullest functioning was being blocked by the lack of planning for extension of care.

In this chapter, concepts which the nurse-educator would hope the nursing student would assimilate and make a part of her frame of reference have been presented. The application of these concepts takes place within the nursing process.

References

1. Levine, S. and Elzey, F.F. A Programmed Introduction to Research. Belmont, California, Wadsworth Publishing Co., 1968.
2. King, Stanley H. Perceptions of illness and Medical Practice. New York, Russell Sage Foundation, 1962.
3. Crowley, D. Pain and Its Alleviation. Los Angeles, University of California School of Nursing, 1962.
4. Socio-Cultural Elements in Case-Work: A Case Book of Seven Ethnic Case Studies, New York, Council on Social Work Education, 1955.
5. Ackerman, N. Psychodynamics of Family Life: Diagnosis and Treatment of Family Relationships. New York, Basic Books, Inc., 1959.
6. Richardson, H. B. Patients Have Families. New York, Commonwealth Fund, 1945.
7. Koos, E.L. The Sociology of the Patient, 2nd ed. New York, McGraw-Hill Book Company, 1954.
8. Willie, C. A success story of community action. Nursing Outlook, 9:19-21, 1961.

9. Black, M. Critical Thinking: An Introduction to Logic and Scientific Method. New York, Prentice-Hall, Inc., 1946.
10. Heidgerkin, L. and Meyer, B. Introduction to Research in Nursing. Philadelphia, J.B. Lippincott, 1962.
11. Dewey, J. How We Think. New York, Heath, 1933.

PART II

The Nursing Process

4

Identifying Nursing Needs

To examine what happens when nursing care is being given is to examine a process, something changing, vital, and growing. Part II is devoted to the description of the nursing process in order to consider what changes take place, not only in the patient but in the nurse—not only in the receiver but in the giver of nursing care.

Hildegarde Peplau[1] defines nursing as a human relationship between an individual who is sick or in need of health services and a nurse especially educated to recognize and to respond to the need for help. The response involves selecting and meeting those needs he or she is able to meet and seeing that other requirements are provided.

Need

What is a need? Kluckholn[2] has defined a need as an unmet requirement (natural or acquired) of an organism that prompts action and is experienced as desire. The self which requires preservation and enhancement is a "bio-psycho-social" being. It requires, therefore, "relatively stable conditions of existence which include not only internal stability as an organism but psychological and social factors which influence *human* stability and the individual and collective actions man may take to establish and maintain relative homeostasis."[3]

In general, homeostasis has been used to refer to the requirement of the organism to maintain an internal stable environment, while the term

39

equilibrium has been used to refer to the state of balance or adjustment to opposing forces and interests which is required to maintain and enhance selfhood. Hans Selye's term for homeostasis, "staying power," suggests a wholeness of the individual which removes the divisions unconsciously imposed when one describes him as a "bio-psycho-social" being.[4] The hyphenated adjective invariably suggests a splitting with the possibility of emphasis upon one attribute to the exclusion of the others. In her poignant description of her own illness, Grace Stuart says, "All damage to the body is first and foremost damage to the self, therefore there is no really good treatment, no scientific treatment which does not take into account the primary necessity for healing and establishing the ego, for making the self picture whole again."[5]

How does the individual human being maintain the state of balance in which he is at ease with his environment? A relatively constant internal environment is provided by circulating blood of such volume and pressure as to meet the changing needs of organs, by an adequate supply of oxygen and nutrition to cells, by fluid and electrolyte balance, by the presence of certain enzymes and hormones, by the maintenance of a definite temperature range, by elimination of wastes, by periods of decreased cellular activity for purposes of repair. In addition, a means of locomotion, the support of body structures, and the protection of soft tissues are provided by a musculoskeletal system. Intact skin and mucous membranes and a reticuloendothelial system protect him from injury and harmful agents. Information about the external environment is provided by the senses of vision, hearing, taste, touch, and temperature discernment, while a functioning cerebral cortex provides the facilities of cognition and association of ideas. Communication with other human beings is provided by speech.[3]

This human being acquires autonomy and independence as he distinguishes between himself and others. He is able to give love, affection, and acceptance to others because he has received love, experienced security, and developed a sense of trust in his earliest experiences with others. He acquires a feeling of self-worth as his role and contributions are recognized in his group experiences. He attains his goals as he acquires the knowledge of the culture in which he lives, and he experiences a feeling of self-fulfillment as he develops his own modes of self-expression. Because he has opportunities to develop long-term perspectives, he relates to larger and larger wholes and sees himself as a part of a universe governed by an infinite purpose.

The optimum state of equilibrium described above is one rarely achieved wholly, and then only for fleeting moments. However, to the extent that one of the requirements is not met, *need* exists and a potential for action is created. When conscious needs are fused, interests appear and goals may emerge. A clue to an individual's needs may often be found in his interests and goals. He prepares for and goes into action to fill those requirements needed to preserve and enhance his being. Thought, feeling, and action are mobilized to help him compensate for the lacks, to adapt to them, to defend himself against the threat they impose, or to put his frame of reference into order.

Needs originate from many sources. Sister Charles Marie, in working out a nursing care formula, describes the patient as made up of a biologic component, individual differences, and a cultural component, within each of which are many variables, some within normal limits, others in excess or deficient.[6] Ruth Freeman reminds the nurse that health needs of the individual and the family may arise from a physiologic condition, from a disease condition so well patterned as to be an entity, from patterns of behavior characteristic of the patient and family, from the sociocultural milieu, or from the external, physical environment.[7]

However, the nurse begins with the person, with what he is and does in his constant attempt to meet requirements. His behavior is her focal point of departure, although knowledge of possible sources of needs supplements the data she assembles from her observation of his behavior. Care must be taken that she does not use knowledge of possible sources of needs to form judgments not firmly grounded on direct observation of behavior.

Behavior as a Manifestation of Need

Behavior is both overt and covert. The former is observable through the use of the senses, while covert behavior must be communicated to another through verbal and nonverbal means. Extrasensory perception is required to become aware of covert behavior. Examples of overt behavior may be found in some of the well-known signs of disease which the nurse notes: pallor, rapid pulse, diarrhea, catatonia, acts of violent aggression, acts of withdrawal from social intercourse, refusal of food, and so on. Covert behavior is made of thinking and feeling or the cognitive and affective components which may not yet be translated into an observable act. Thought and feeling are often conveyed through words but even more expressively through the inflection of the voice, the facial expression, the gesture, the posture of the body, the rate of movement, the tread of the foot. The communication of thought and feelings brings the nurse most closely to what the individual is: "As a man thinketh in his heart, so is he."[8] On the other hand, the act is the fruition of thought and feeling and makes man truly knowledgeable to man: "By their fruits ye shall know them."[9]

Observation of behavior, then, is the key to identifying needs and determining what requirements for self-realization and stability are lacking. Observation is a method of collecting data and assembling evidence to be used for an established purpose. Observation not only involves the reception of sensory stimuli but also the perception of the individual observer. *What* the observer sees, feels, smells, touches, and hears is determined by his phenomenologic field, his frame of reference which has been created by the organized, integrated meanings of his life experiences. Observation can therefore never be wholly objective. It is highly selective; sensations are received, ignored, distorted, or transformed within the observer's private world.

Observation of behavior accomplishes its purpose when as complete evidence as possible is assembled and when relationships between parts of the data can be readily demonstrated. There is a clear distinction between what can be grossly observed and what is communicated. Overt behavior which is manifest can be observed. Covert behavior has to be communicated. Headache, pain, a sense of fullness, grief, or anxiety are communicated to the observer when sharing, a kind of revealing, takes place between the observer and the observed. Perhaps this communication is the extrasensory perception needed to observe covert behavior.

The nurse is often very skillful in observing overt behavior. Frequently her earliest nursing experience is one in which emphasis is placed on noting signs, particularly vital signs of temperature, pulse, and respiration. Other observable signs of the organism's response to internal and external stimuli are blood pressure; color of skin and mucous membrane; amount, kind, color, and odor of excreta; range of motion of a limb; muscle contraction; salivation; and so on. Unfortunately she too often knows so thoroughly the signs associated with a disease entity that she approaches the diabetic, cardiac, or arthritic patient with a well-formulated mental list of expected behaviors.

Mr. A. who has diabetes may meet none of the nurse's expectations but may manifest other highly significant overt behavior. If she can temporarily shelve her checklist and perceive Mr. A. as unique, she may be able to see relationships between his sleeplessness, his overacting, his silence when his family visits, and the limping gait which appears when he walks down the empty corridor. To observe the unexpected and to make new associations between parts of the collected data is to be the skillful observer. If the nurse can be aware of her "mind set," her "blind spots," she is more apt to surmount them and discover new data and new relationships.

The Illness Experience

In discussing covert behavior and how it is communicated, it may be well to review some of the cognitive (thinking) and affective (feeling) components of the illness experience. What comes to mind at once? Very probably the reader selects loneliness, pain, aches of all kinds, anxiety, fear, guilt, resentment, grief, and despair. He recalls, too, the ignorance (lack of specific knowledge), the misunderstandings, the beliefs bred into him about the efficacy of certain kinds of treatments, the significance to him of an ambulance or an oxygen tent. These are the thinking and feeling parts of illness which are covert and must be communicated to an observer.

If observable manifestations of pain were listed, physical behavior might include perspiration, clenched hands, wincing movement, restlessness, crying, blinking, sudden change in color. Social behavior runs the gamut of silence, flippancy, avoidance of people, garrulity, attention demanding, complaining. But manifest social behavior requires interpretation. Sharing and exploring must take place between the patient and nurse so that interaction is set into motion. In this way only can there be the revealing of the personal frame of reference and the meaning of pain to the individual. How the pain feels, where it is located, how long it lasts, what other sensations accompany or initiate it—all this must be shared and explored by the nurse and patient.

What prevents this sharing and exploring? Illness or dis-ease means some degree of imbalance; the individual is not at ease with or in command of himself and his environment. Something must be done to restore balance. This he may be able to do for himself or someone must assist him, even take over completely those things he has formerly done for himself. Illness and a degree of dependency go together, but dependency is not wholly acceptable. It may bring great comfort to the patient, but the innate urge to handle his hurt himself is part of human nature. The patient, then, hesitates to share. He often marshals his defenses, uses those patterns of flight, fight, and passivity which have served him before in his attempt to take care of matters himself.

Closely allied to this ambivalence about dependency are three other obstacles to sharing. One is the patient's image of a good patient and of what is expected of him. A good patient may be one who "can take it," who takes what is given him but never asks, who causes the physicians and nurses no trouble. This image is rooted in the family experiences of illness when the child is early taught that men don't cry, that one does as he is told when he is ill. It is so often reconfirmed for the individual as he hears nurses exchange remarks about the patient who never cried out during a painful dressing, who has "never once had his light on." On the other hand, the individual may perceive the patient as one who asks for and is given attention, who expresses fully his wants, who is expected to show his pain and discomfort. An elderly lady, following the removal of a cataract, groaned and moaned loudly to the great distress of her family. Finally, one member asked, "But, Grandma, does it really hurt?" The woman answered, "Of course not, but I thought this was what I was supposed to do."

Again, one shares when he can reasonably expect that what he shares will be received and used. In strange surroundings, with a strange nurse, the patient may have no previous experience in this identical situation to guarantee that the nurse will help him if he does share. True, he may have found other nurses receptive and helpful in another experience, but this is a new, truly unique experience, and until trust is established, he is wary. The author, as a patient over many weeks, has noticed this experimental period as new patients are admitted to a four-bed ward. Sometimes the patient carries on a running exchange of pleasantries, or answers only in monosyllables, or even apologetically asks for a forgotten piece of equipment in the bedside stand. This initial behavior is a decided contrast to that of later days when he has become engaged in the joint task of restoring his health. Hildegard Peplau describes this stage of nurse-patient relationship as one of orientation, the period in which direction is sought by "feeling-out."

A final obstacle to sharing may be those expectations which the patient brings with him from other illness experiences which were referred to in the previous paragraph. He may expect the nurse to be technically skillful, efficient, and well-organized, with many demands made upon her by many people. He may bring with him the image of the nurse as the warm, gentle person who soothes and comforts and is ever near him.[1] He may see the nurse as his avenue to the physician, the person who carries out the physician's plan for him, someone who has been told and in turn tells him what he must do. Frequently, the nurse is seen as someone who keeps the wheels going, who is responsible for his new environment. When the patient is at home, he often sees the nurse as a resource person with an uncanny faculty of knowing what is useful and available to him in the community.

But sharing involves the nurse as well as the patient. She, too, has thoughts and feelings prompted not only by what her senses convey to her but by previous experiences or situations related to the immediate one. Her observations lead to reports of the patient's condition as "comfortable, disagreeable, distended, or well-nourished," or his attitude as "disoriented, stupid, angry, or pleasant." These are immediate interpretations of what has been conveyed to her through many media of communication. She arrives at these interpretations through some kind of association and differentiation which is the outcome of her perception of behavior. What she saw or heard stimulated thoughts and feelings from the repository of all her experiences. Perhaps she is uncomfortable with disagreeable people; perhaps she cannot tolerate stupid people; perhaps angry patients make her angry, too.

Dr. Samuel Liebman discusses the physician's immediate reaction to and personal attitude toward the patient. He writes of the intern called to see an old man who had been brought into a county hospital in a comatose condition, terribly dirty and crawling with lice. In the patient's history, the intern wrote, "This patient is filthy dirty and is crawling with lice. I will examine him as soon as he is properly cleaned and de-loused."[10]

The nurse has ideas, too, of what "a good nurse" should say and do. A good nurse does not show anger. She should like all patients and be able to work with all families. She works quickly, gets her tasks done, and so organizes her work that she economizes on both time and effort. It is "unprofessional" to care or give of one's self too much. The good nurse is well-informed, accurate, and logical in her response to inquiries or questions.

Sylvia Bruce, in her account of a study of the reactions of nurses and mothers to still-births, cites comments by nurses which reveal the nurse's concern that she must have an answer, some verbal solace to give:[11] "You can always say God has his reasons and we must have faith ... If there is no reason for the death, what *is* there to say?" One nurse told the mother she was lucky she had two at home and time for more. One would conclude that nurses felt something must be said so that their feelings and those of the patient could be controlled. The mothers' comments were: "I was so lonely, I wanted to talk to anyone about anything. ... I couldn't care about what God thought—I only knew how I felt. ... This baby was important at the moment, not the ones I had had or could have. All you think about first is what you don't have. ... Some nurses were nice enough. They worked fast and looked busy. They did whatever you asked but efficiently, quickly, and left."

The nurse brings to the patient her reactions from other situations which have not been resolved or left unabsorbed, and these block or prevent communication between nurse and patient.[12] If the nurse has not felt free to question a head nurse's directive or challenge an instructor's interpretation of another situation, she carries out the directive or uses the interpretation in the immediate situation without exploring the appropriateness of the former or the validity of the latter. Her ability to communicate with the patient, and thereby help meet his need, is impaired.

The nurse has beliefs, values, codes of behavior, and attitudes which affect her reaction to how another mourns, how he manages pain, faces bodily disfigurement, meets pending death, responds to birth. She and the patient, as human beings, are alike in their search for meaning, their search for selfhood.[13] If she is unable to recognize, face realistically, and explore *with others* her own anxiety, loneliness, guilt, and other states of distress, she comes to the patient unprepared for the exploration necessary to meet his needs.

This linkage of self with others has perhaps never been more beautifully expressed than by John Donne, the English poet:

No man is an island entire of himself; every man is a piece of the continent, a part of the main, if a clod be washed away by the sea, Europe is the less, as well as if a promontory were, as well as if a manor of thy friends or of thine own were; any man's death diminishes me, because I am involved in mankind; and therefore never send to know for whom the bell tolls; it tolls for thee.

Devotions, XVII, 1624

Whatever may be the blocks of communication which may lie within the patient and the nurse, it is the responsibility of the nurse to initiate communication to start the chain of interaction which will reveal each to the other in terms of what are the patient's needs and how can the nurse help meet them. This exploration begins the nursing process. The nursing skills essentially involved are those of observation and communication.

The Face-to-Face View

Much has been written about the interiew as a method of exchanging information and gaining insight into another's thoughts and feelings. The interview has been called a conversation with purpose. Perhaps this description inadvertently places emphasis upon conversation. *Entre nous* is a face-to-face view or look and implies the use of all the senses of the observer and the observed. Most often in nursing, the face-to-face view occurs in a situation in which acts of ministration are being carried out or are expected by the "interviewer." This factor distinguishes the nurse-patient interview from the interview between the teacher and student, social worker and client, employer and employee, and even the physician and patient.

To the nurse who is preoccupied with what she does for and to a patient, the element of doing is a major block to observing and communicating. She is much too busy with doing. To the nurse previously oriented to the desired outcome of the face-to-face view, namely, the gathering, testing, clarifying, and organizing of data so that she may gain insight and identify needs, the act of ministration becomes a vehicle or conveyor of her interest, her concern, and her caring for another person. The act of ministration requires the use of all the nonverbal media at her command. The pressure she uses in rubbing a back, the rate of her movements in the room, the way she looks at a patient, the inflection of her voice when she answers a question, the position she takes when the doctor changes a dressing, the care she uses in handling personal possessions, the time she takes to listen to or just be near the patient, the loosening of covers at the foot of the bed as she passes by, the turning of a pillow or placing a bed where the patient can get a view of a budding tree or one laden with snow—all these acts convey the way she perceives the patient and is relating to him. The setting of the usual nursing situation in many ways lends itself more easily to expressing care and concern than does the office desk and chair, or the round conference table which other professional workers use. The interviewer has the opportunity to observe overt behavior, the action which tells her much.[11]

The dynamics of the nurse-patient interview may best be described as the process of perceiving and relating to another human being in such a way as to communicate concern, respect, empathy, compassion, and sympathy.[14] These feelings are initiated by the nurse so that they may be translated into action directed towards meeting the health needs of the patient. A single word *rapport*, is often used to describe this particular relationship. Rapport is established when the nurse and the patient have worked out mutually acceptable roles in which each is comfortable and knows what is expected of her and what she can give to the other. Because this relationship requires emotional involvement of each participant, the nurse, as the initiator, must understand feelings, be aware of why they exist, and use them purposefully, not only to reinforce the relationship, but to translate them into action. If the ultimate purpose of the relationship is kept in mind, then the nurse will not find herself entangled in other kinds of human relationships.

The free, mutually giving and receiving relationship of friendship and love is not equivalent to the helping and being helped relationship of the nurse and patient.[15] Rapport may progress into the patient's interest in the nurse as a person, into emotional dependence upon the nurse. Since love and hate are intimately related, the nurse may find herself the recipient of either when the professional relationship has gotten out of hand. Miss Fenlason[15] has described other processes in the helping interview: accepting behavior, reducing hostility, meeting resistance, avoiding and easing tension. Tension is often used constructively in helping another person reach a decision. Actually, each of these processes is an integral part of building the helping relationship.

What sets these processes into action? What keeps them going? Often the nurse gropes for something to say. It has been implied that action language is often most expressive. A conversation may be initiated by: 1) Letting the patient take the lead when this comes naturally; 2) Commenting on something you have observed; 3) Using a general opener—for example, to a mother at a Well Child Conference, "How do you manage? Do you get any help?" In many situations, the lead has been taken by the nurse in action, and the patient finds it safe and comfortable to talk first. Commenting on something observed begins the testing and exploring to which the nurse must subject all her observations and then the act of listening begins. The "general opener" must be sufficiently personalized for the patient, lest he hear only a pleasantry which spells rejection of what concerns him most at that moment. A well-intended "How are you this fine day?" often closes the door for a patient who contrasts himself and his own aches and gray sky to the attractive young nurse whose step is buoyant and color high. He thinks, "What would she understand of how I feel on this unbright day?"

Whatever the beginning, the nurse must find ways to become the listener. To listen actively and creatively means listening with eyes as well as ears, with one's mind and heart. It means wanting to hear more, recognizing that much has been left unsaid, that there are significant omissions, inconsistencies, and recurring themes.[16]

Helen Creighton and Sister Gabriella Richard write of a ten-year-old boy with tetralogy of Fallot and his need to talk about his fear that he was outgrowing his heart.[17] The nurse squarely faced with him the fact that people do get scared, that people do sometimes run away from what scares them. She implied that she was there to help him when she said, "When people stick together to face something that threatens them, they often do find ways to help each other." But this led to his answer, "Misery ain't always got company." Little by little, the nurse began to grasp the significance of the behavior she observed: the cold, purple-hued little hand that dug finger nails into her arm as he said, "I have to stop growing!"; the low, serious tone; the slow leaning forward towards her. At every point, she strove to keep the boy's line of thought developing. What she heard, she and others used to allow him to have some active part in managing or working with his fear.

Many techniques of listening have been described. One method is the questioning repetition of end phrases which may invite further elaboration of what has been said. A statement by the interviewer of what he believes the interviewee is really feeling or thinking may lead to clarification, confirmation, or denial. A nod or verbal signal often conveys the nurse's acceptance of a behavior pattern which the patient constantly tests; he must make sure that he is not being judged as to rightness or wrongness, that he will not be told too soon what to do—in short, he is testing his "safety."

Unfortunately, nurse-patient interviewing techniques may be used without the giving of one's self. With an increasingly well-informed public, the technique without the personal concern is easily recognized, and no interchange occurs. Form and substance can be clearly distinguished. Phrases such as "Tell me more," or "How do you feel about it," or the reflective response can become habitual, but the interviewee responds to the whole person, not to the phrase alone.

Since one of the purposes of the nurse-patient interview is to exchange information, questions are used frequently. Questions may elicit a "yes" or a "no," or they may invite more sharing, opening many avenues to pursue. Such open-ended questions tend to keep the interviewee talking. A double-barrelled question, requiring two answers or provoking two unrelated responses, is nearly always unproductive. When the question implies confidence and faith in another's willingness to work with those who are trying to help him, the patient recognizes the trust invested in him and responds accordingly. "Were you able to drink your eggnog?" implies the only deterrent is his ability to swallow or to tolerate fluids. "Why" questions may be perceived as probing or requiring a reasoned and reasonable answer. When feelings are intense, "why" should be avoided. Too many questions may structure an interview too much, and many significant tangents are lost. In general, the information the interviewee selects on his own initiative to present, in an order and sequence he evolves, is more revealing of his thought and feeling than the information called forth by an orderly series of questions structured by the interviewer.

In some situations, history-taking is the nurse's responsibility. In others, she makes use of the history taken by the physician, the admission officer, and others to complement her observations. She adds to the history as she gains further information in her face-to-face contacts with the patient. History-taking implies that the purpose of the interview is to gather information concerning a sequence of events leading to, or the circumstances associated with, the patient's present situation. Often a record form specifies the information to be sought: for example, age, residence, current occupation, onset of the illness, signs and symptoms which were noted, previous illness, previous pregnancies, type of delivery, when enuresis began, what was happening in the family when enuresis began, and so on. The actual taking of a history affords an opportunity for patient and nurse to review objectively a sequence of events or a set of circumstances in the course of which perspective is gained. If questions are not asked too rapidly, if they are asked warmly and with interest, with an extra comment by the nurse, more significant information is often given in the response. Ruth Freeman[7] refers to the nurse who, in taking the ages of children as she begins a family health record, comments, "You had to wait a long time for John to come along, didn't you?" Miss Freeman speculates on what might be called forth: "Yes, he's certainly spoiled by all of us," or "Well, we really didn't plan to have John but now that he's here we are glad." Factual information has not been increased but some glimpses of a family's life history have been gained.

Something should be said of the choice of words in an interview. Words carry connotations or auras which may call forth negative or positive feelings. Words are often labeled "bad" because sufficient evidence has been gathered to indicate that a chain of negative reactions is begun when the word is used. For example, the word "terminal" carries with it a finality that precludes any further effort. Paul H. Brauer, in discussing the use of the word "terminal" with families, points out that the implication is that the patient is already dead and "the victim should immediately be stricken from the records," particularly if the disease is cancer.[18] He suggests substituting words like "severe," "advancing," or "progressive," which emphasize "quality and process" and do not magnify the element of time.

Words also connote social class and, because they are foreign to the listener's culture, make people strangers to each other. Within professional groups, a jargon is developed out of a highly specialized vocabulary; the patient exists outside this inner sanctum and must cope with words and phrases he cannot question. An interesting exercise is to keep a list of words and phrases which are perfectly familiar to the "insiders" or health team, but which are ambiguous or unknown to the "outsiders" or general public. The practice of using simple words which express clearly what is meant could well be encouraged in all professional groups. Illustrations and analogies which make use of the professional groups.

Illustrations and analogies which make use of the patient's experiences are helpful. A thrombus explained by an analogy to a clump of sticks and weeds around which the water must flow at the edge of a lazy stream would have some meaning to the patient from a rural community but none to the city dweller; double parking in a main traffic artery would help the latter visualize the narrowed lumen of a blood vessel.

Methods of Developing Observation and Communication Skills

Thus far, observation and communication have been discussed as the means by which the nursing process is initiated and data is collected, interpreted, and evaluated for the evidence they present of nursing needs. How does the nurse develop observation and communication skills? If she has experienced or is experiencing with her head nurse, supervisor, or instructor the kind of warm, accepting relationship which has been described in the preceding paragraphs, she will be more nearly able to communicate acceptance, concern, and warmth to patients. To experience rapport as one who is being helped, gives far greater meaning to that term than does the most eloquent description found in a book or heard in a classroom. Feelings are learned by experiencing them. Likewise, action language as well as somatic language is learned in the presence of other persons.[19] The inexperienced nurse sees the patient relax with a skillful message, fall asleep after skillful turning, weep with relief when the nurse slips quietly into the room after a painful dressing. Participating in a situation where nursing skills are used successfully to meet human needs makes unavoidable the improvement of communication skills.

An observation chart or an anecdotal behavior record written during the early days of a patient's admission and at later intervals may be used as a tool to improve gross observation. However, care should be taken to separate observations from the observer's interpretation of the behavior. The anecdotal behavior record should describe overt behavior noted in a variety of circumstances: for example, at meal time, after visiting hours, during a treatment, with a physician, with a visiting teacher, and so on. The single anecdote should include a brief description of the setting, the circumstances, what was said or done, listing only the sensory receptions of the observer. Interpretation and evaluation of the incident is then summarized separately by the observer and shared with a skilled observer. Occasionally, interpretation and evaluation of the single incident is written as a footnote to the anecdote. In both the observation chart and the anecdotal behavior record, the observer is attempting to review her observations as objectively as possible and to recognize the involvement of herself in what she perceives.

One of the best methods to gain insight to interaction and the communication process is the process-recording which may be taped or written. The advantage of taping is the opportunity to recall orally an experience with a patient, without the distortions which often occur when one writes of a situation in which one's self is under scrutiny. In either the written or taped process-recording which is recorded in retrospect, much is deleted, changed, and elaborated, since the factor of selection (remembering what one wants to remember) is great. However, what one recalls is significant, and with a third indirect observer, the more skilled nurse, clues unrecognized or forgotten by the student can be pointed out. Process-recording of interaction with the same patient or the same family over an extended period of time has proved so helpful to the nurse that in some agency situations (chiefly public health nursing agencies) she is asked to intersperse her more brief and structured recording on the clinical chart or family record with a process-recording of a home visit or a day with the patient in the ward unit. The nurse is often able to see movement in the interaction, to see where further exploration was necessary to really identify a need, to become aware of what blocked the patient's recognizing his need, and to evaluate the action she took in terms of involving the patient's participation.

Role-playing can be used when the nurse is ready for group help. She may not be comfortable with this method, feeling she subjects herself to criticism, even a little fearful of what role-playing may reveal. Often simplified role-playing is a good starting point. A staff nurse may relate an impasse reached with a patient. After a discussion of the problem, it may be suggested that she play the role of the particular patient and another member of the group become the nurse. After a few minutes, each may be asked how she felt and to what she responded negatively or positively. The situation can then be discussed by the group once more. More elaborate role-playing involves briefing the characters of their roles and a warming-up period; this helps the players understand their roles more clearly. Care must be taken to preserve spontaneity and to cast the characters so that a role having unfavorable characteristics is given to someone with sufficient group status and personal security to carry it successfully.[20] The action is halted when there is a natural closing, when enough behavior has been exhibited for group analysis, or when the players have reached an impasse.[20] Group analysis focuses on what understandings gained from the role-playing can be applied to the problem situation. A summary of what the group has learned is then helpful. On occasions, a replaying may be used to test group recommendations for change in action.

Data helpful to identifying health needs can be obtained by other means than direct observation and communication. The family record and the clinical record will give age, occupation, marital status, family members, residence, and nationality. The disease diagnosis, the parts of the body involved, the symptoms presented by the patient and family to other health workers, the events which precipitated the onset of illness are to be found in records and reports. Conferences with co-workers, and particularly with the family, will amplify what has been directly observed and communicated. If conferring with the family can be done in the home setting, data can be gathered about the social and cultural setting of the patient as well as the health potentials of the family. Factors which predispose the individual to illness, or which may operate to perpetuate it, can be observed.

The observation of the patient's behavior and the communication between the patient, his family, and health workers, yield data which can be used to define his health needs and to select appropriate action. The nursing process begins with a personal relationship in which "two persons come to know and to respect each other as persons who are able and yet different, as persons who share in the solution of problems."[1]

References

1. Peplau, H. Inter-personal Relations in Nursing. New York, G.P. Putnam's Sons, 1952.
2. Kluckholn, C. Culture and Behavior: Collected Essays. New York, Free Press of Glencoe, 1962.
3. Nordmark, M. T. and Rohweder, A.H. Science Principles Applied to Nursing. Philadelphia, J.B. Lippincott, Co., 1959.
4. Selye, H. The Stress of Life. New York, McGraw-Hill Book Co., 1956.
5. Stuart, G. The Private World of Pain. London, Allen & Unwin, Ltd., 1953.
6. Frank, Sister Charles Marie. Viewing the patient from the stratosphere. Nurs. Outlook, 11:62-65, 1964.
7. Freeman, R. Public Health Nursing Practice. Philadelphia, W.B. Saunders Co., 1957.
8. Proverbs, 23:7.
9. Gospel of St. Matthew, 7:20.
10. Liebman, S. Stress Situations. Philadelphia, J.B. Lippincott Co., 1954.
11. Bruce, S. Reactions of nurses and mothers to still-births. Nurs. Outlook, 10:88-91, 1962.

12. Orlando, I. The Dynamic Nurse-Patient Relationship. New York, G.P. Putnam's Sons, 1961.
13. Jersild, A.T. When Teachers Face Themselves. New York, Bureau of Publications, Teachers College, Columbia University, 1955.
14. Travelbee, J. What do we mean by rapport? Amer. J. Nurs., 63:70-72, 1963.
15. Fenlason, A.F. Essentials in Interviewing. New York, Harper, 1952.
16. Garrett, A. Interviewing: Its Principles and Methods. New York, Family Welfare Association of America, 1942.
17. Creighton, H., and Sister Gabriella Richard. When you are scared. Amer. J. Nurs., 63:61-63, 1963.
18. Brauer, P.H. Should the patient be told the truth? Nurs. Outlook, 8:672-676, 1960.
19. Davis, A.J. The skills of communication. Amer. J. Nurs., 63:66-70, 1963.
20. How to Use Role-Playing. Leadership Pamphlet No. 6, Adult Education Association of the U.S.A., 1960.

5

The Nursing Diagnosis

Process and Product

The term *diagnosis* may be used to refer to a process or to the outcome of that process. The failure to make this distinction has led to much confusion and an initial rejection of diagnosis as a part of the nursing process. Whenever facts are carefully investigated for the purpose of determining the nature of a thing, diagnosis is taking place. When the parent examines the factors in the home situation which seem to precipitate or set the stage for the child's temper tantrums, he or she is engaged in the act of diagnosing. The lawyer who makes an inventory of the presenting evidence is making a diagnosis. The facts he works with and the outcome of his investigation are very different from those of the physician or the parent, but the process he moves through is the same. Facts are assembled; factors in the situation are considered; relationships and association are established; an appraisal is made; and a judgment reached.

The nurse in the act of diagnosis observes, communicates, tests her findings with the patient, further confers with the family and her co-workers, reviews experiences with other patients, searches the scientific bases of symptoms observed, and identifies the patient's needs. Her assessment of the patient's dis-ease and what the dis-ease means to the patient becomes the nursing diagnosis. What she has done parallels the physician's act of examination, observation, history taking, laboratory testing, conferring with other physicians and health workers, referring to the literature, and eventually arriving at a medical diagnosis or the statement of a disease entity or entities.[1]

The medical diagnosis leads to a therapeutic plan, a *design for cure* which is primarily concerned with supplying what is lacking. The nursing diagnosis leads to a *plan for nursing care* which is primarily concerned with sustaining, preserving, and conserving the individual's adaptive, defense, and enforcing mechanisms, and with removing or reducing stress or stimuli. The nursing care plan also includes measures related to the plan for cure (the application and execution of the legal orders of the physician), but its uniqueness resides in its focus upon nursing therapy, those measures directed toward the alleviation of the patient's dis-ease and the modification of his perception of his illness.

The distinction between cure and care is not an artificial one; nor can it be ignored. Someone has pointed out the difference between the comments: "I have been home *nursing* my cold" and "Tonight I am going to *doctor* my cold." In the first instance, the individual has consciously used factors in his environment (internal and external) which reinforce and make possible the operation of his own defense and reparative systems. Increased fluids, bed rest, warm moist air—these and other environmental factors are used according to patterns of care he has experienced in his own family. He "copes" with his cold. In the latter instance, external aids not normally a part of the individual's environment are used. He "medicates" himself, relying on past cure experiences or the persuasiveness of advertisements which describe treatment and cure. He "treats" his cold. Care is essentially custodial, supportive, and educative in nature while cure is remedial.

As the nurse observes and communicates with the patient and family, needs become apparent. This data must be sorted and weighed. Which of these needs can be met by nursing care? Which of these can be related to the functions of other health workers? Which of all the needs apparent to the nurse are recognized by the patient, which by the family? This sorting, weighing, and referring is an appraisal which leads to the statement of the nursing diagnosis. The criterion always applied reads: "Is the need which is recognized or felt by the nurse, the patient, his family, or by the nurse alone one which requires the help of the nurse?" If the answer is yes, then the need is a nursing need and will be used in determining the nursing diagnosis.

In the interval during which the act of diagnosis takes place, the more the patient is involved in the investigation of facts and the appraisal of findings, the greater is the assurance that the nursing diagnosis will be a valid one. The inclusion of the patient in the exploration of what is needed preserves his selfhood and helps him to relate to others during the highly self-centered experience of illness. When the nurse is engaged in diagnosing the nursing needs of a family group, she again explores with them and involves them in the formulation of the nursing diagnosis. Even when the patient is acutely ill or the family group disrupted and disorganized, in imbalance, the nurse seeks ways to develop their recognition of their needs. Often she herself makes a *tentative* nursing diagnosis, arrives at an impression comparable to the notation often found in the early entries the physician makes in the clinical chart before a medical diagnosis is confirmed, but she continues to seek verification from the patient and family. The illness or dis-ease, the nature of which she is trying to determine, requires continuing investigation shared by the patient and family.

A Definition of the Nursing Diagnosis

In the preceding paragraphs, the term *nursing diagnosis* has been used repeatedly. An attempt has been made to make its meaning clear by describing the act of diagnosing. However, because there has been some resistance to the use of the term *diagnosis* in nursing practice, the reader will find a wide variety of terms used to label the product of diagnosing. Terms such as nursing assessment, nursing problems, nursing needs, nursing care objectives, as well as nursing diagnosis have been used. Abdellah and co-workers[2] listed 21 nursing problems which some readers have challenged as statements of major nursing needs. Others have contended that these are statements of nursing care objectives. Whatever term is selected, its meaning must be clarified if there is to be a common understanding among those who use it.[3] Nursing diagnosis, as used in this volume, can be defined as "an evaluation or assessment, based upon verifiable data, of an individual's state of dis-ease and what that dis-ease means or signifies to him in his life situation." Within this definition is the term dis-ease, a state in which the individual is not able to function his best or to live his fullest.

The identification of nursing needs requires a sorting out of those needs which can be met by nursing care and those which require referral to other sources of help. Observation of and communication with the patient and family lead to an assessment or evaluation of assets and liabilities, strengths and weakness, in the patient's or family's condition and life situation. Out of the nursing diagnosis emerge nursing care objectives or goals. Nursing action then becomes directed towards removing the obstacles to reaching the nursing care goals. The obstacles are nursing problems specifically related to the nursing care objectives. Graphically the progression is as follows:

Needs   Nursing Needs   Nursing Diagnosis
Nursing Care Objectives   Nursing Action to Remove Obstacles

Perhaps some distinction should be made here between a need, a demand, and a want. To want and to need are not synonymous; however, what the patient wants or desires is highly significant and may provide important clues to needs. The craving for a highly spiced, high caloric dish from home is often indicative of the need for some symbol of family concern. The patient who wants a warm pillow support when she lies on her side may be expressing a need to maintain muscle relaxation by avoiding strain and chilling. The desire must be taken into consideration, as it involves the will to have and indicates drive. The patient who demands is expressing a drive to attain not always what he truly needs but some kind of an end. This drive is a part of motivation which, when directed towards a goal, is essential to the business of regaining and maintaining or improving health.

An estimate of the patient's and family's competence to meet nursing needs is a prerequisite to formulating nursing care objectives. For some nursing needs, the patient's physical ability, his knowledge, his attitudes will be adequate. For others, the nurse must supply the requisites until the individual's adaptive potentials have been realized. The family's competence to meet nursing needs must be appraised in terms of their knowledge of the disease condition, their motivation, their application of good health practices, the physical environment of the home, and their use of intra and extra family resources.

An appraisal of the individual's and family's ability to meet nursing needs and a prognosis of expected change (an estimate of adaptive potentials) serve to establish priorities and to define immediate and long-term objectives of nursing care.

Two interesting studies have been made to rate or measure the ability of the individual and his family to meet nursing needs as well as their adaptive potentials. The patient profile described by Mary Edna Williams[4] is " . . . an ability and behavior scale built on the assumption that behavior and ability can be observed and rated, and ratings used constructively in planning patient care." Seven nursing needs were selected and the patient's physical ability to meet the nursing needs for nourishment, elimination, rest, exercise, social interaction, safety, and therapy was rated as adequate, less than adequate, or inadequate. The patient's observable response to these seven nursing needs was rated as showing positive interest, a passive response, or an extreme response. His response, which might be described either as organized behavior with goal-directed activities, as no observable interest in meeting the need but accepting of nursing care, or as extreme response in either a positive or negative manner, served to give a clue to his motivation and therefore to his potentials for developing the ability to meet nursing needs. Such a patient profile in written form could be a helpful tool in arriving at nursing care objectives and in determining the nursing prognosis.

The second study, described by Ruth Freeman and Marie Lowe,[5] is concerned with " . . . improving the quality of nursing judgment of family competence and in developing a systematic method for stating family competence in areas generally accepted as falling within the province of community nursing." Certain "elements" basic to family and community nursing practice were identified, such as "physical independence, therapeutic independence, knowledge of the condition, application of principles of general hygiene, attitudes toward health, emotional competence, family living, physical environment, and use of community resources." These elements can be recognized as requirements which must be met if the family in the illness experience is to remain a self-sustaining, balanced group who will use the illness experience and its own resources to reinforce and further develop its strengths as a group—in short, to achieve, maintain, and further family health.

A rating scale from 0 to 9 was devised, with provision for the nurse to substantiate by her observations the rating given. At the same time, a rating scale was used to scale the anticipated competence level at the end of nursing service or at the end of three months. The latter served as a prognosis of change in family competence or ability to meet its own illness needs. Thus the family's starting point and its expected achievement served as a guide which the nurse could use in estimating to what degree nursing care and nursing service might have effected the change in family competence.

Appraisal of the individual's or family's ability to meet nursing needs or to respond to needs with initiative and direction requires a developed skill. Evidence of the ability to meet nursing needs independently can be acquired through skillful observation in the home setting. In the hospital setting, appraisal of the family's ability is more difficult, but it can be judged with a fair degree of accuracy when members of the family are given an opportunity to participate in the patient's care. The trends to provide for family involvement in pediatric and maternity hospital units are encouraging. Appraisal of the individual's ability is possible if the patient, insofar as he is physically and emotionally able, is given an opportunity at every turn to share in decision-making, to care for himself, and to measure his own progress.

The Statement of Nursing Care Objectives

Nursing care objectives are stated in terms of the desired changes in the behavior of the patient and his family—changes in the patient's physiologic behavior, his psychologic behavior (thinking and feeling), and his psychomotor activities. The goals may indicate that the nurse carries the responsibility for effecting the change or that she will help the patient or family effect the change. The following examples of nursing care objectives illustrate the emphasis upon what the nurse must do for the patient or upon what change in behavior she will help the patient and family achieve. The nurse has as her goal:

To maintain an adequate oxygen supply for Mr. Simon.
To help Mrs. South understand the relationship between fatigue and muscle spasm.

To help Mrs. Russell feel more at home on the ward unit.
To help Mrs. Maxwell recognize and report to the physician signs and
symptoms of cardiac embarrassment.
To protect Mrs. Lane from falling.
To assist Marcia in developing the ability to communicate verbally with
others.
To help the Brown family provide safe play facilities for their two
preschool children.

Even when the stated goal indicates that the nurse carries the
burden of responsibility, it nevertheless requires that the patient use his
resources to the utmost. The achievement of any nursing care objective,
whether it be concerned with physiologic or psychosocial behavior,
requires the active involvement of those in whom the change is to
occur. To bring about this involvement requires creative nursing.

Some nursing care objectives are more immediate than others. It
will be remembered that in the assessment or evaluation of the
individual's condition and his life situation certain priorities were
established. Those priorities may be found in the immediate nursing
care objective. Again, goals which are mutually acceptable may be more
quickly attained, and the satisfaction which success brings further
motivates the patient and family. The mother may be most eager to
recognize her infant's demand-feeding pattern. Once she has succeeded
in reaching this goal, she is ready to consider immunizing the infant
against certain communicable diseases. The nurse constantly considers
how realistic the nursing care objective is in terms of the patient's and
family's acceptance of it and their readiness to make the desired change
in behavior.

It may be helpful now to retrace the steps actually taken in arriving
at a nursing diagnosis and in setting up immediate and long-term
objectives of nursing care for a real patient, Mrs. Katherine Sullivan.*
An observation record of the patient's behavior, with an interpretation
of nursing needs, a statement of the nursing diagnosis, and immediate
and long-term objectives of nursing care, follow a description of Mrs.
Sullivan and a history of her illness up to the time of her admission to
Hospital X in January of 1962.

*The material concerning this patient, including observation chart and analysis of
nursing needs, has been taken (with some elaboration) from the records written by
a nurse who cared for her.

Mrs. Sullivan grew up in Massachusetts and was graduated from a finishing school. She very much wanted to become a nurse but her parents did not approve. Many years later, at the age of 55, she studied practical nursing. She received ceritification and a license to practice, but never did so.

She was married at the age of 18. She had five children, three of whom died in the first few days of life, from what she described as hemorrhage. One daughter died a year ago from "grief over the death of her husband." The other daughter is married and lives out of town.

For the past 25 years, Mrs. Sullivan has owned and operated her own beauty salon. She lives alone in a second floor apartment of a two-family house in a residential area of the city. Her companion for 13 years has been a much loved parrot. This bird died two days after Mrs. Sullivan entered Hospital X.

In 1950 Mrs. Sullivan noticed increasing thirst. She went to her family physician who told her she had diabetes mellitus. She was instructed in self-administration of insulin but was not restricted in any way as to diet. Her diabetes was kept under control by 36 units of regular insulin in the morning and 34 at night. Shortly thereafter, she noticed the aches and pains in her legs became progressively worse. A burning sensation in her thighs often kept her awake, and her only relief was to walk about. Six years ago, pains in the calves of her legs became so severe that walking a short distance was impossible and her working hours, with much long standing, were distressing. Numbness in both feet occurred soon after rising, with marked loss of sensation in her right foot. In late December, she went to her physician who ordered hospitalization for diagnostic tests. She entered Hospital X in January of 1962.

A medical diagnosis was made of arteriosclerotic occlusion of the right femoral artery. A bypass graft was made of the right femoral and popliteal arteries. Later a thrombosis of the arterial graft of the right femoral artery occurred and gangrene of the right foot developed. A mid-thigh amputation of the right leg was done. Later stump repair was necessary.

Miss Martin, the nurse who cared for Mrs. Sullivan throughout much of this period, wrote the following "patient portrait."

Mrs. Sullivan is a warm, outgoing person. She is devoutly religious and frequently reads her be-thumbed Bible. Her clergyman visits her frequently, and each greets the other cordially.

Mrs. Sullivan is meticulous in her personal habits and is very conscious of her own personal appearance and that of her roommates. She is never super-critical but expresses the wish that she could make others comfortable and attractive.

A record of observed behavior was kept during one week, with an interpretation of the nursing needs demonstrated.

DATE	NAME: Mrs. Katherine Sullivan OBSERVATIONS MADE	SIGNATURE	NEEDS WHICH CAN BE MET BY NURSING CARE
3-12-62	(Day of operation-repair of the stump) Frankly states fear of operation. Says she fears anesthesia will not be wholly effective, that she will awaken before suturing is completed. Talked with anesthetist yesterday but seems not satisfied with what she was told. Refused to read morning paper which she usually does; read prayer book all morning. Referred to only living daughter for first time, "She is very busy with her church work."	H. Martin	Protection from eternal injury. Acquisition of further knowledge; some meaningful association of ideas about anesthesia and surgery. Time for spiritual meditation.
3-13-62	(1st postoperative day) Mrs. Sullivan cried briefly in the early A.M. because of pain in her right thigh. Refused		Relief from pain. Help in turning.

3-14-62		
	to turn because she feared pain would increase. After medication, she combed her hair, read her mail, greeted visitors (former employees). Refused breakfast and lunch but took fluids including fruit juice.	Adequate intake of nutrients.
		H. Martin
3-14-62	(2nd postoperative day) Mrs. Sullivan's sense of humor has returned. Bathed herself this A.M., changed position as needed, saying, "I know that to move about is good for me." She applied light make-up, chose gaily-colored pajama top, ate good breakfast. Called nurse for roommate whose condition worsened this morning.	Feeling of self-worth.
		H. Martin

Date	Notes	Signature	Goal
3-14 (continued)	Later expressed concern lest the dressing adhere to wound when physician dresses it. Spoke of possibility gangrene may "set in" in her other foot because prior to hospitalization the circulation in left foot was poor. She talked with physician today about this worry.	H. Martin	Protection from harmful external agents.
3-15-62	Face drawn and haggard this morning, but more active physically. Moves about in bed easily and gives herself all of daily care. Complains the early morning insulin injection interrupts her early morning sleep. Is glum, withdrawn, not talkative, though obviously trying to be cordial with other patients in room. Is tense, apprehensive of the dres-		Adequate amount of sleep. Satisfying social interaction.

67

sing which she expects physician to do today. Eyes filled with tears several times this morning though she has not cried openly.

H. Martin

NURSING DIAGNOSIS

Mrs. Sullivan is a warm, outgoing, devoutly religious person; she has frequent contact with her clergyman. She is very concerned about the comfort of her roommates and does all that she can to help them. She has a good sense of humor and understands the need for exercise in bed and for prevention of injury to the remaining lower extremity. Circulation to the left foot is badly impaired. Her occupation has required long hours of standing and walking. Her appetite is poor, and she is very apprehensive lest she lose her other limb. She lives alone and has one living daughter whose residence is out of town.

IMMEDIATE OBJECTIVES OF NURSING CARE

1. To help Mrs. Sullivan adapt to and live with pain.
2. To help her understand the relationship between adequate nutrition and wound healing.
3. To help her prepare for weight-bearing.
4. To help her maintain circulation in the left lower extremity.
5. To help her express anxieties, fears, and concerns for her future.
6. To explore with her resources in her personal world.

LONG-TERM NURSING OBJECTIVES OF NURSE

1. To help Mrs. Sullivan achieve independence in ambulation and in self-care.
2. To help her accomodate to her limitations and modify her living and work arrangements.
3. To help her prevent further circulatory impairment.

Notice that the immediate objectives are goals which Mrs. Sullivan had indicated were her own and which she is now ready to try to attain. The objectives state changes in behavior (thinking, feeling, doing) which can be demonstrated in overt behavior. Immediate objectives are compatible with long-term ones and will contribute to the attainment of the latter.

A parallel example may be found in the study of the Mason family. Here the nurse was able to identify the family's nursing needs, to establish a nursing diagnosis and to set up objectives of nursing care.

Mr. and Mrs. Mason, aged 24 and 20 are a Negro couple with a baby son born five months ago. The young couple live with Mr. Mason's father and mother in a very poor neighborhood. Mr. Mason, Senior, is a minister, as is his wife's father. Mr. and Mrs. Mason, Senior, have a two-year-old adopted son. Mr. Mason, Junior, has a history of asthma, for which he is now receiving medical care. He is a window cleaner but is frequently unemployed.

Mrs. Mason was admitted to the services of the public health nursing agency in her eighth month of pregnancy, having been referred from the prenatal clinic at the local hospital. She had reported there to have her pregnancy determined but did not return until her eighth month. She feared going to the hospital and only on the insistence of her mother did she go to the hospital to be delivered.

Labor was long and difficult, lasting 24 hours. Mrs. Mason was heavily sedated and remembers little, except that there was some discussion of a cesarean section. She did not see her baby in the hospital. The postpartum period was uneventful and she was discharged after a postpartum examination at the end of six weeks. Later she developed a glycosuria. She reported that she eats constantly but is losing weight. Menses are irregular and she expresses great anxiety lest she have more children.

The baby has developed several allergies; among others, he is allergic to eggs, cereals, juices. At the age of one month, he was admitted to the hospital for bronchial pneumonia. In another six weeks, he was admitted for an upper respiratory infection and an otitis media.

During the nurse's visits, Mrs. Mason talks of feeling very inadequate in caring for the baby and in keeping house. She has had four months of preparation for practical nursing. She often says she thinks the baby is handled too much, that he should have been in an incubator in the hospital. She is tense in handling him, very serious in manner and speech. The nurse identified family health needs and supported her conclusions with observational evidence:

NURSING DIAGNOSIS

The nurse selected the major health needs to be a feeling of emotional adequacy and sustaining family relationships. The former was recognized and accepted by Mrs. Mason and there was some indication that individually, if not as a group, the family recognized the latter need.

This is an extended family with medical care provided by hospital clinics and the hospital emergency room. The young mother has had four months of preparation as a practical nurse. The elder Mason couple support their daughter-in-law.

Mr. Mason, Junior, has a history of asthma. The infant son, 5-month-old, is allergic to eggs, cereals, and juices, has had bronchial pneumonia and otitis media, and was hospitalized for upper respiratory infection before the age of three months. Mrs. Mason, Junior, has a glycosuria and loss of weight. She is tense in handling the baby, fearful of future pregnancies, and expresses feelings of inadequacy and even

OBSERVATIONS MADE

1. Mrs. M. talks of feeling inadequate. Tense in handling baby. Shows indecision in care of baby, often expresses, "I should have done differently." Father rarely mentioned and then in terms of his trying to find work. Mrs. M. wishes no more children.

2. Mrs. M. did not receive prenatal care until 8th month. Afraid of hospital; had hospital delivery only because mother insisted. Baby taken to emergency ward without previous medical care in home. Baby not taken to Child Health Conference regularly.

3. Mother has erroneous ideas as to pattern of growth. Compares baby's developments with events in history of adopted 2-yr.-old which mother-in-law relates. Family diet very poor; high in carbohydrates.

4. Mr. and Mrs. M. do few things together; his parents disapprove of his "idleness" and say "we thought he would do better after he married the right girl."

5. Stairs are rickety. Rooms smell of oil from space heater. Buildings are close; the only sunny courtyard littered with rubbish. Provisions for preserving food limited to very small, noisy, partially operating electric refrigerator.

FAMILY HEALTH NEEDS

1. Feeling of emotional adequacy. Security in handling infant.

2. Medical supervision for family.

3. Knowledge of child growth and development.
   Balanced, nutritious family diet.

4. Sustaining family relationships.

5. Healthful physical environment.

guilt. The young Masons do few things together. The housing is poor, stairs unsafe, heating and ventilation poor, and refrigeration of food inadequate.

IMMEDIATE OBJECTIVES OF NURSING CARE

1. To help Mrs. Mason gain confidence in caring for her baby by helping her apply what she had learned in the practical nurse course,

and by helping Mrs. Mason, Senior, give more responsibility for homemaking to her daughter-in-law.

LONG-TERM OBJECTIVES FOR NURSING CARE

1. To help the family develop competence in the use of medical supervision and care.
2. To help Mr. Mason, Junior, assume the father role. Helping the family modify its physical environment might later be possible if some degree of family adequacy could be achieved in terms of meeting the needs of individual members.

Summary
Conclusions

What changes have taken place in the nurse's phenomenologic field as she moves through the process of diagnosing? She considers what she knows of the patient and his family, what this knowledge means in terms of health and nursing needs, what more she needs to know. She sorts and weights these collected data, giving priority to some and tabling others until they can be further confirmed or amplified. She locates areas of potential movement, areas of sufficient discomfort to the patient and family to make action acceptable. In what direction should movement occur? Which goals are immediate and realistic? What changes in the family's and patient's behavior can be expected if the goals are attained?

This chapter has described a way of thinking, an approach which is based on a diligent study of human behavior and which leads to an ever-increasing comprehension of the breadth and depth of nursing care.

References

1. Chambers, W. Nursing diagnosis. Amer. J. Nurs., 62:102-104, 1962.
2. Abdellah, F., Boland, I., Martin, A., and Matheney, R. Patient-Centered Approaches to Nursing. New York, Macmillan, 1961.
3. Little, D. and Carnevali, D. Nursing Care Planning. Philadelphia, J.B. Lippincott Co., 1969.

4. Williams, M.E. The patient profile. Nurs. Res., 9:122-124, 1960.
5. Freeman, R., and Lowe, M. A method for appraising family public health nursing needs. Amer. J. Public Health., 53:47-52, 1963.

6

The Planning of Nursing Care

Whenever an attempt is made to describe a process, the risk is taken of seeming to outline a series of orderly steps. A process is dynamic, not static, ever-changing with all its components interrelated. These interrelationships imply that change in one component effects change in all other components. The collection of data continues, the assessment of those data is on-going, and the nursing diagnosis changes with new insights. Planning is concerned with how to attain current goals, both immediate and long-term, but it is always subject to the influence of a reassessment of the patient's and family's state of dis-ease and to the revision of goals. Planning includes not only a choice of action but the evaluation of the consequences of that action as well.

Kinds of Nursing Care

Since planning leads to action, it may be helpful to group nursing activities in terms of the kinds of nursing care required to meet the patient's needs. In other chapters, it has been pointed out that nursing care is concerned with 1) helping the patient preserve and sustain his own defense and ordering mechanisms, 2) supplying what is needed for remedy or repair, 3) helping him learn new ways of living or restoring himself to a balanced state, and 4) helping him prevent injury, infection, or disease. Some needs require supportive or sustaining nursing care; others, remedial or curative nursing care; still others,

TABLE 1. Functions of Nursing Care

In Accordance with Patient's Needs	Related Activities
Giving supportive nursing care.	Turning patient every hour. Giving hi-caloric between meal nourishments. Serving hot, black coffee before breakfast is served. Giving demerol, 75mgm,p.r.n. for pain.
Giving remedial, curative nursing care.	Preparing patient for operative procedure. Irrigating colostomy every morning. Irrigating Foley catheter once a week. Injecting intramuscularly a daily antibiotic.
Giving reeducative nursing care.	Teaching patient to take small frequent feedings. Helping family to plan rearrangement of sleeping quarters for patient with cardiac decompensation. Teaching patient to use walker. Instructing patient and family as to sources of information concerning prosthesis, dressing supplies, etc.
Giving preventive nursing care.	Instructing patient before surgery how to breathe, cough, turn, and use a trapeze. Demonstrating how to apply elastic bandages to aid venous circulation. Teaching the pregnant woman relaxation exercises. Helping parents learn developmental needs of infant during the first 6 to 8 weeks of life. Helping parents anticipate growth and developmental patterns of the preschooler. Helping family prepare for progressive changes in long-term illness of a family member.

or restorative nursing care. With the concept of health as a dynamic changing state of being and serving, preventive nursing care is recognized as a fourth category of nursing care.

Bundles of nursing activities directed toward similar kinds of nursing care are called functions. Table 1 gives examples of nursing activities related to giving supportive, remedial, reeducative and preventive nursing care.

The Choice of Action

The innumerable nursing activities which could be listed leads to the central question of what governs the choice of action. Because the healing arts have their origin in the curative, remedial care of the sick, nursing activities have in the past stemmed from the medical care plan and medical therapy; thus, the major choice of action has not been the nurse's choice. However, judgment leading to choice was exercised by and delegated to the nurse when she chose to give a medication with or without fruit juice, to instill a solution at a specific temperature, or to use a certain kind of equipment. In recent years it has been recognized that the nurse, because of her intimate and continuous contact with the patient, best knows the patient's idiosyncrasies, his ability to help himself, his strengths, and his motivations. It can no longer be ignored that comprehensive nursing care requires of the nurse independent judgment and choice of action to sustain and reeducate individuals and families so that their ability to help themselves regain, maintain, or promote health may be restored or developed to its fullest extent. The independent planning of nursing care is best illustrated, then, in carrying on the function of giving supportive, reeducative, and preventive nursing care. However, the interdependence of all planning toward the health care of people is inevitable. As this chapter focuses upon the nurse's choice of action, the reader must be aware of the basic assumption that the nurse's choice is always compatible with and related to the planning of other members of the health team. Part III will be devoted to methods of working with others to effect the coordination and evaluation of health care plans for the individual patient and family.

Nursing Care Principles: How They Evolve

Selecting appropriate action may be likened to the search for tentative solutions in problem-solving. A reassessment of a situation, A, leads to the identification of factors which are similar to those in other situations, B, C, and D, in which a nursing action has occurred. The consequences of that action are recalled and are compared with the outcomes desired in the present situation A. The steps which led to the choice of action in situations B, C, and D are reviewed. Factors are examined as variables which might change the outcome. If common denominators in situations A, B, C, and D are sufficiently great and the risks which the variables impose not too threatening, then a decision may be made to take the nursing action which was employed in situations B, C, and D.

Sometimes no similar situations can be found in one's own previous experience. The experience of others is sought by way of professional literature, clinical records, or consultation. The same comparing, contrasting, matching, cross-matching, and isolation of variables takes place.

From experiences, generalizations are made which are used again and again as guides to action; these are frequently called principles. When a principle evolves from a controlled laboratory situation in which the testing of hypotheses has led to sufficient proof to establish an operational truth, it becomes a scientific principle. In other words, a principle may be based solely upon experience or upon experimental data *and* experience. A scientific principle is accepted and used as a guide to action as long as it demonstrates its validity in experience.

In a brilliant lecture on "The New Style of Science"[1] Henry Morgenau reminds us that "science harbors no final, absolute truth," and that "axioms turned into postulated, basic hypotheses are maintained as long as they agree with the facts of experience." "Man's facts are turned into acts, and the feedback between the knower and the known makes old commitments absurd when new evidence is submitted." Morgenau recounts the meaningful story of the youth who ventured to lift the veil over the picture entitled *Truth*. "Did he not see," says Morgenau, "Dismiss your quest for truth in final formulation and embrace the greatest human virtue, called Quest for Truth."

Much emphasis has been placed in recent years upon the teaching of scientific principles of nursing care. Students have been quizzed on "underlying principles" and have produced statements of "shoulds" and "oughts" which is as undependable as guides for the choice of intelligent action as are the rote recitation of the steps in a procedure. Perhaps the emphasis should be shifted to helping the learner develop those concepts essential to the decisions she makes in giving nursing care.

In his perceptive attempt to dissect the concept of stress, Hans Selye[2] describes the effort involved in abstracting from facts "some common hold on many of them, through which they can all be coordinated to a common point." In this manner concepts are formulated. As they develop, the personal frame of reference is changed, comprehension is extended, and finally action is effected. With today's rapid increase in knowledge, there is an urgency to pull facts together, to find some common links and to develop concepts from which hypotheses can be formulated, put to test, and the resulting generalization applied to action. Hans Selye writes, "Whenever a large number of facts accumulates concerning any branch of knowledge, the human mind feels the need for some unifying concept with which to correlate them. Such integration . . . is also practically useful. It helps one to see a large field from a single point of view . . . in order to ascertain where more detailed exploration of the ground would be most helpful for its further development."[2]

One of the major tasks of teaching today is selecting information which may help the learner to understand the basic concepts under scrutiny. A principle is meaningless unless a thorough analysis has been made of the concept which it tests. For example, the concept of pressure as a force used to circulate fluids (blood and lymph) and, thus, related to cell nutrition is made up of such observed facts as:

1. Fluids flow from an area of higher pressure to one of lower pressure, and the rate of volume flow is directly related to the pressure gradient.
2. The contraction of skeletal muscles propels the lymph in the main thoracic duct.

3. Expansion of the lungs upon inspiration exerts a pressure upon the main thoracic duct, forcing lymph onward.
4. The descending diaphragm upon inspiration compresses the contents of the abdomen which exert a pressure on the abdominal vessels. This causes lymph to flow into the main thoracic duct from the abdominal lymphatics.
5. The amount and kind of blood in the superficial blood vessels affects the color of skin and mucous membranes.

The concepts of pressure and cell nutrition, when used by the observer of human behavior, have developed into a major principle of homeostasis which Nordmark and Rohweder[3] state as follows: "The blood serves as a means of transport for substances to and from the cells, and the volume of and pressure of circulating blood must be maintained within certain limits to provide for changing demands of the organ."

These concepts are used to formulate a principle of nursing care; namely, when there is a possibility of a large quantity of blood pooling in the periphery and/or the splanchnic region, a rapid fall in blood pressure can be expected. The nurse uses this principle as she selects the action to be taken. She may apply an abdominal binder or elastic stocking, she may change the patient's posture very gradually, or she may carefully avoid high temperature in preparing the bath. She discontinues the application of heat or cold if the skin changes are extreme and persistent.

The nurse uses another principle in the measurement of blood pressure: pressure beneath the free surface of a liquid is equal to the vertical height of the liquid times its density. The basic concept again is pressure. The underlying fact is that arterial pressure can be measured by equalizing the external pressure applied against an artery with the pressure within the artery.

Another example from Nordmark and Rohweder[3] deals with the concept of fluid balance, a subconcept of homeostasis. The observed facts include:

1. The isotonicity of body fluids is maintained largely by the retention and elimination of water and certain electrolytes primarily, sodium and potassium, and is regulated by kidney function.
   A) A loss of sodium is followed by loss of water.
   B) The ingestion of sodium is followed by water retention.

C) The state of hydration of cells depends primarily upon the concentration of sodium ions in the extracellular fluid.

2. Normally, the body's fluid output balances the intake except when new tissues or fluids are being formed. Fluid is then retained.

3. The amount of tissue fluid varies with:

A) The filtration rate of fluid from the capillaries. This in turn varies with:
  1) The rate of blood flow (an inverse relationship).
  2) The capillary blood pressure (a direct relationship).
  3) The osmotic pressure of the blood (an inverse relationship).
  4) The capillary dilation (a direct relationship).
  5) The concentration of sodium and proteins in the tissue fluid (a direct relationship).
  6) The concentration of oxygen in the blood (an inverse relationship).

B) The return of fluid from intercellular spaces into the blood. This in turn varies with:
  1) The patency of the lymph channels (a direct relationship).
  2) The rate of blood flow (a direct relationship).
  3) The pressure of the lymphatic fluid (an indirect relationship).
  4) The concentration of sodium and proteins in the plasma (an inverse relationship).

4. The volume of urine secreted varies with the amount of glomerular filtration and the amount of tubular reabsorption.

A) The amount of glomerular filtration varies directly with:
  1) The amount of filtering surface.
  2) The blood pressure in the glomeruli.
  3) The amount of renal blood flow.
  4) The rate of tubular absorption.

B) The amount of glomerular filtration varies inversely with the osmotic pressure exerted by plasma proteins.

C) The amount of tubular reabsorption of water varies directly with:
  1) The water content of the blood.
  2) The amount of antidiuretic factor produced in the posterior pituitary.
  3) The amount of adrenal cortical hormone secreted (because of the effect on sodium loss and potassium retention).
  4) The blood level of estrogens.

D) The amount of tubular reabsorption varies inversely with:
  1) The rate of blood flow in the efferent capillaries.
  2) The concentration of threshold substances in the tubules (e.g., glucose).

The nurse who has a grasp of the concept of fluid balance uses as her guide the principle that measured intake and output are a reliable index to fluid balance. She measures the contents of a container into which fluid drains from a tube inserted into the body. She reports polyuria and frequency, and she expects them when the patient is cold, when he is emotionally upset, when he is receiving diuretics, when there is hypoactivity of posterior pituitary gland, and so on.

Hans Selye[2] has developed the concept of inflammation as reaction to injury. Connective tissue cells and fibers; red and white blood cells in the blood vessels; their response to the irritant which has been demonstrated microscopically or which is observable to the naked eye; the cause of the redness, heat, swelling, pain, and dysfunction; the benefits and detriments of inflammation—these are some of the facts which make up the constellation of ideas known as inflammation. Perhaps the most basic fact concerns the regulation of inflammation by the pro- and anti-inflammatory hormones, the production of which is stimulated by the adrenocorticotropic hormone (ACTH) and the somatotropic hormone (STH) secreted by the pituitary gland.

Should therapy aid the inflammatory reaction to injury or inhibit it? The answer depends largely, so Dr. Selye says, "on the nature of the aggressor"[2] (the irritant or invader). If the aggressor is dangerous and further invasion of the body is highly undesirable, then aiding an inflammatory response is the choice to make. If the aggressor is harmless, then inflammation is not helpful and should be inhibited. This principle helps in making the decision whether to apply heat or cold.

The concept of behavior may be explored as a function of the relationships between identifiable antecedents. The concept of culture can be seen as accepted channels through which individual needs can be met. The observer must determine what factors have been linked together to form the coordinated concept of behavior and culture. This interrelated concept is one of the determinants of individual behavior patterns. Principles formulated from this complex concept have helped the nurse select the appropriate action in dealing with such situations as the young mother who resists the post-partum examination or the elderly couple who refuse hospitalization of one member.

The criteria which the nurse may use in selecting the action to be taken are:

1. Are there underlying principles which can be used? What concepts

do these principles represent? What facts which make up that concept
are in evidence in this particular situation?
2. How predictable are the desired outcomes if the action being
considered is taken? Is the prediction based upon my own past
experiences, upon the experience of those who are experts, or upon
generalizations based on experiment as well as experience?
3. Will I be able to identify the results which are the direct outcomes
of this specific action, or are there many variables in the situation
which cannot be controlled?
4. Is the action being considered feasible in terms of available
resources (personnel with necessary skills), materials, and time?
5. Is the action compatible with actions required to give other kinds of
nursing care? (Will preventive measures, such as turning and exercising
in bed, negate other measures instituted to conserve strength?)
6. Does the action provide for as much patient participation and
self-help as he is capable of giving?

Criteria 2 and 3 deal with a very important element in judgment
and decision-making: estimating results or weighing possible and
probable consequences. Actions are part of a continuum and therefore
have antecedents as well as consequences. Because the nurse has
observed the patient's skin become red with continued pressure, she can
predict that with the added insult of continued moisture, the skin will
break down with the further use of a rubber air-ring. She will choose,
then, to turn the patient frequently, exposing the skin to air and dry
heat. Because the patient took fluids after careful mouth care, the nurse
concludes that mouth care with an emollient and astringent at regular
intervals is a necessary nursing activity. The nurse must observe the
consequences of the nursing care presently being given and evaluate it
before selecting subsequent action.

AVAILABLE RESOURCES

The well-known criteria for the appraisal of a nursing procedure
include economy of time, materials, and effort, as well as the comfort
and safety of the patient and the therapeutic effectiveness of the
procedure. Any choice of action must take into consideration the
amount and kind of skill required to carry out the action. Some courses
of action may require skills which the nurse does not possess. It is the
wise nurse who considers her ability to carry out successfully a course

of action before she undertakes it herself. The suctioning of secretions from the mouth and oropharynx when a tracheotomy has been performed may require a technical skill she does not possess. The nursing action is an imperative one. Her course of action is to secure help and supervision at once.

Not only does the nurse consider her own resources in terms of abilities and skills but she assesses those of the patient and family as well. The patient may have considerable health information, the family may know a great deal about the disease condition of a family member, a child may have developed considerable muscle coordination. These are resources which the nurse must also use in selecting her course of action.

Priorities are determined by the nurse who is aware of the time and effort involved in an action. Pulling tight and smooth a wrinkled drawsheet and patting the skin dry under a perspiring, cyanotic patient in an oxygen tent may be the best choice when nursing time must be divided between three critically ill patients in the same unit. Action which will prevent progress of the disease process or which will relieve stress takes priority over other ministrations, since the length of time the individual organism must cope with a disease agent or stress is related to the duration of resistance and the rapidity of fatigue.

RELATIONSHIP OF THE ACTION TO
A UNIFIED HUMAN EXPERIENCE

Obviously, the same patient or the same family may need several kinds of nursing care. Human needs do not present themselves in categories. During the illness experience, the whole range of nursing care—supportive, remedial, reeducative, and preventive—is required. However, the patient and family are single entities, and the synthesis of nursing care requires a constant awareness of the response to all areas of nursing activities. Giving an analgesic before dressing a surgical wound or giving a back rub and mouth care before administering a soporific are examples of planning a sequence of nursing activities which reinforce each other. Giving an irrigation with the same equipment to be used in the home is an example of carrying out an activity concerned with remedial care in such a way that reeducative nursing care is supported.

All kinds of nursing care are interdependent. Remedial nursing care is directly dependent upon the medical therapeutic plan. Therefore, the nurse must weigh carefully the consequences of a nursing activity with respect to the total therapeutic plan and its objectives. The patient sees no distinction in the purpose of the various kinds of care he receives. All nursing care to him symbolizes the care and concern he has for himself. In planning her nursing care activities, the nurse must consider the significance of her activities to the patient. Do they make sense? Do her actions seem to contradict each other? At the end of the day, does the patient feel there has been concerted action directed towards helping him get well, or has it been a series of unrelated events seemingly having no thread of common purpose except to get the day's work done? The task of coordinating activities, synthesizing phases of health care, and giving continuity to the action of the many individuals concerned with the care of the patient requires group planning and decision-making.

INVOLVEMENT OF PATIENT AND FAMILY
IN DECISION-MAKING

Nursing care is directed towards helping the patient and family meet those needs which they cannot supply alone, by exercising the skills characteristic of nursing—ministering, observing, communicating, counseling, teaching, and administering. Developing the self-help ability of the patient and family is also part of nursing care. An ability unused deteriorates. Illness, because of the dependency it creates, imperils the patient's self-help ability. Only by encouraging its use within the limits of the illness situation can the nurse hope to avoid its deterioration. Selecting action which requires the patient to participate or which brings about the desire to help is therefore important.

To arrange the surroundings so that the patient can give himself personal care may be more time-consuming for the family or the nurse. It may mean to the nurse a less tidy patient unit, a less cleansing bath, a less well-groomed patient, or it may even deprive her of the personal satisfaction of having her care preferred by the patient or family. The nurse must examine the amount of patient participation she allows in both planning and giving care. This may reveal to the nurse what factors she uses as guides to her choice of action.

HOW THE DECISION-MAKING ABILITY MAY BE DEVELOPED

Does the nurse have freedom of choice? Are not the physician's orders to be carried out? It is true that decisions as to medical therapy are not the nurse's own decisions. But the nurse alone exercises judgment as to how orders are to be carried out. She implements the medical care plan and helps evaluate its effectiveness. She must choose to whom to teach good health practices; when, what and how to teach in what settings; what measures to institute to conserve strength, to aid or inhibit the local defenses of inflammation, or to prevent injury or infection; and how to orient a patient and family to a hospital experience. What approach does the nurse use with the patient who must give up smoking because of cerebrovascular disease? Does she ignore his use of tobacco? Does she explore with him the effects of smoking, the measures he might take to stop smoking, and the improvement he could expect? Does she frequently express to him her faith that he can give it up? She alone governs the choice of action. Is she not free to decide to use a footboard, a cradle, or pillows to relieve pressure upon the lower extremities? Can she not choose to emphasize vitamins B and C in helping a patient select his diet, in helping a family plan a weekly menu? Does a nurse ever, independently of a physician's order, measure intake and output?

In spite of the fact that for many years the existence of nursing orders has been recognized as authentic, rarely does one find nursing orders on the patient's order sheet. Nurses have selected an action often without conscious use of criteria, frequently on an empirical basis. They have observed the consequences of their action and passed on to other nurses what actions seemed to have worked. However, no appreciable advance has been noted in the organization of facts and concepts or in the formulation of hypotheses from clinical laboratory experience. Without deliberate, thoughtful selection of action, nursing care can never be evaluated for its own worth.

To help the nurse examine what guides she uses in planning nursing care, it has been suggested that she review nursing measures which are used in situations where the patient has, for example, intractable pain, incontinence, disorientation, loss of consciousness, aphasia, and so on.

She lists these measures and opposite each states under what circumstances she would use the measure and for what reason or reasons. This approach is suggestive of Cyril McBride's *Signs and Symptoms,* in which presenting signs and symptoms are reviewed as to possible causes and subsequent general treatment. Because of her orientation to procedures, the nurse may be more comfortable with an approach in which she reviews familiar actions such as injection, instillation, irrigation, application, insertion, again for the purpose of examining alternatives and determining what guides her choice of action.

Evaluation of the Outcomes of Nursing Intervention

The continuous evaluation of the results of the nurse's actions provides the basis from which generalizations or principles eventually emerge. The study of overt and covert behavior through observation and communication now focuses upon evidence of change due to the nursing measures employed. The nurse must ask what signs indicated the change, what change has taken place, and what caused the change.

The change in behavior which the nurse seeks is the desirable change or improvement, a movement toward health or equilibrium. The dilemma she encounters is one occasioned by the "absence of any reliable information concerning predictable responses of patients and no agreement as to physiological and psychological responses which can be judged good or bad."[4] Some patient welfare measures were used in experiments at the State University of Iowa Hospital.[5] These have been defended as sensitive to change and indicative of difference between individual patients when control and experimental groups of patients were used. Some of the scaled measures used were mental attitudes, physical independence, mobility, skin condition, patient's opinion of nursing care given him, and the physician's evaluation of the patient's condition and progress. Patient's activities comprised another group of measures: time spent in bed, in a chair, up, communicating with others, and in occupied leisure. Finally, certain clinical measures were used: number of hospital days, fever days, and postoperative days, doses of narcotics, analgesics, and sedatives. All of these are general indices of patient welfare that can be used for groups of patients but are not appropriate for estimating the individual patient's response.

The observation and evaluation of the individual patient's behavior in terms of improvement still need to be greatly refined. Laurie M. Gunter[6] points to three major aspects of disease which may have to be considered in evaluation of the patient's reaction to illness. These are 1) the disorder of the function responsible for his symptoms, 2) the pathologic processes of anatomic structures and organs, and 3) the psychologic reactions of the patient to these disorders and pathologies. Change in each of these areas may need to be considered separately, but total response, in the final analysis, must be considered if the individual's welfare is to be evaluated.

To relate desirable change to its cause or causes is not possible until more is known of the human organism's ability to adapt to stress and the means of aiding that adaptation. Change in behavior, however, can be estimated, and associations can be made between the nursing care given and changes in the behavior noted. This evaluation involves judgment and therefore runs the risk of being influenced by the evaluator-observer's bias and opinion. The observer may find it wise not to predict how he thinks the patient will react, but to "observe carefully and see if a pattern emerges."[4] Descriptions of the patient's behavior are far more helpful than such generalizations as "improvement in attitude," "less anxious," or "moderate regression." From an aggregate of such descriptions, rating scales may be developed which are useful when groups of patients are being studied. When descriptions of patient's reactions can be given in quantitative terms—such as, so many patients developed cracked nipples, so many played with their toys when parents left after visiting hours were over—the error due to observer's bias can be controlled.

Evidence of the results of many nursing activities related to remedial nursing care seems easily obtained and even quantitatively measurable. The pulse rate slows following digitalization, temperature is reduced after an alcohol sponge, urine output is increased after the moist application of heat to the abdomen, and intraocular pressure decreases when an antimiotic drug is administered. Change can be stated in exact terms of before and after an action, with relative, if not absolute, assurance that the specific change noted was due to the nursing activity. Unless it is possible to repeat the sequence of events with all elements within the series unchanged save for the nursing activity, the question can still be raised as to what exactly caused the slowed pulse rate, the reduced temperature, the increased urine output, or the decreased intraocular pressure. Since somatic behavior is part of the total response to total environment, even physiologic change cannot be associated directly with a single cause. "Patient response may be due to the disease process itself, to the therapeutic program, or to interaction with any or all of the persons who participate in therapy."[4]

When change in psychosocial behavior is being evaluated, it is far more difficult to associate cause and effect directly. As a supportive measure, the night nurse chose to look in frequently on the patient who often signaled for trivial requests or even signaled "by mistake." When she found the patient awake, she asked him to put on his bathrobe and stroll down the hall with her. On the third night, she noted his light was never flashed and he slept soundly throughout the night. This change continued the remainder of the week until the eve of surgery. Could she be sure that her action had caused the change? Was it the minister's visit during the day, improved ventilation during evening relief hours, the nonthreatening events of the preceding hospital day, or simply acclimation to hospital environment. No control of the myriad elements in the situation is possible, and the nurse has no positive assurance of the effectiveness of her treatment.

Some interesting studies have been reported of nursing approaches or nursing activities used with patients placed in experimental and control groups. Such a study was made by Rhetaugh Dumas and Robert C. Leonard on the effect of nursing on the incidence of postoperative vomiting.[7] The nurse-investigator spent one hour with the patient before surgery, went with him to the operating room and remained with him until he went on the operating table. In two of the three experiments, the nurse took care of the patient in the recovery room, ending her contact with him when he returned to the ward. The nurse explored with the patient her observations of his behavior to determine whether he was experiencing distress, what was causing it, and what was needed to relieve the distress. She used the information she gained to select an appropriate action to relieve the distress and checked with the patient to learn whether this course of action did relieve his distress. With the total of 51 gynecologic surgical patients participating in the study, the incidence of postoperative vomiting was lower among the experimental group. Further research supported the conclusion that nursing care directed towards relieving the emotional stress prior to surgery does relieve postoperative distress.[7]

A preliminary report[8] has been made of an experimental study at Walter Reed Hospital of patients with pressure areas and decubitus ulcers. Hydrogen peroxide cleansing, followed by packing the cavity with granulated sugar and applying a dressing for 24 hours was tried. Other methods such as the topical protective spray, the alternating pressure mattress, light therapy, and various types of support have also been studied. The continued systematic study of the behavior of groups of patients who have or have not experienced a selected nursing measure or approach may lead, in time, to nursing prescriptions as reliable as medical prescriptions. The individual's reaction to nursing therapy may become more predictable.

The planning of nursing care involves the choice of appropriate action based upon established criteria and the continuous evaluation of individual and group response to nursing care. Deliberate thoughtful selection of the nursing action with the desired change in patient behavior ever in mind, makes possible the evaluation of the quality of nursing care. With greater insight into the significance of individual behavior, there will be greater assurance of finding the relationship between specific nursing action and desired change in the patient.

References

1. Morgenau, H. The new style of science. Yale Alum. Mag., Feb., 1963.
2. Selye, H. The Stress of Life. New York, McGraw-Hill Book Co., 1956.
3. Nordmark, M., and Rohweder, A., Science Principles Applied to Nursing. Philadelphia, J.B. Lippincott Co., 1959.
4. Quint, J.C. Delineation of qualitative aspects of patient care: Discussion by Rosella Schlotfeldt. Nurs. Res., 11:204-206, 1962.
5. Aydelotte, M.R. The use of patient welfare as a criterion measure. Nurs. Res., 11:10-14, 1962.
6. Gunter, L.M. Notes on a theoretical framework for nursing research. Nurs. Res., 11:219-222, 1962.
7. Dumas, R.G., and Leonard, R.C. The effect of nursing on the incidence of postoperative vomiting. Nurs. Res., 12:12-15, 1963.

8. Verhonick, P.J. Preliminary report of a study of decubitus ulcer care. Amer. J. Nurs., 61, 1961.
9. Herzog, E. Some Guidelines for Evaluating Research: Assessing Psychosocial Change in Individuals. Washington, U.S. Department of Health, Education, and Welfare, 1959.

7

The Nursing Care Plan

The nursing plan is a design in which actions are organized into some kind of sequence and progression. It has some degree of permanency. It will be carried out by more than one nurse and will be shared, not only by those who implement it but also by others who give health care to the patient and family. Therefore, the nursing care plan should be written and accessible to those who care for the patient and family. It is readily available as a kind of blueprint for action. It must be flexible enough to allow for revisions, additions, or deletions.

The Purpose of a Nursing Care Plan

The form of the nursing care plan must reveal the purpose of planning, that is, the nursing care objectives. These were developed from an exploration of health needs which required nursing intervention. A nursing diagnosis was made, and long-term and immediate nursing objectives emerged. Nursing activities related to supportive, remedial, reeducative, and preventive nursing care were selected to be carried out in an ordered pattern. The effect of nursing activities upon the patient were observed and evaluated. The culminating points in the planning process must appear in the nursing care plan if it is to be a record of the total nursing care picture.

The Observation Record

The nursing care plan does not replace the written record of the nurse's observations of the patient's and family's behavior and her exploration and interpretation of that behavior in terms of nursing needs. Nursing notes also include an account of changes in behavior as well as the nurse's assessment of those changes in terms of progress towards mutually acceptable goals. These notes and observations are a vital part of the clinical record, as they reflect behavior and record interaction with and response to the total environment in which therapy is being undertaken. The nurse's notes which simply state the medications and treatments given, with cryptic evaluations of behavior such as "more comfortable," "less anxious," or "slept well" without evidence are valueless as an aid to planning. Consequently, the nurse whose notes are ignored, regards the time spent in writing them as worthless.

Writing notations of behavior and the interpretation of its significance in revealing nursing needs requires skill which is acquired by guided practice. The form itself may help the nurse focus upon the purpose of recording behavior. Two parallel columns, one given to an account of behavior (interaction and response), and the other to periodic interpretation of the meaning of that behavior, may be more helpful than a blank form. The nurse's notes read by and shared with another more experienced nurse, often take on new significance to the writer and she becomes aware of omissions, judgments made too hastily or based on bias and opinion without sufficient evidence and clues to patient reactions. The nurse may gain the insight which can be expected from a true process recording. Some nurse leaders, interested in the improvement of public health nursing service, have recommended that the nurse periodically write a process recording of the interval spent in the home with the patient and family. Such a recommendation might well be considered in the hospital situation to develop the nurse's comprehension of the role of perception and feeling in the observation of patient behavior.

VARIATIONS FOUND IN DIFFERENT SETTINGS

Perhaps it is here that a comparison should be made between the records related to nursing care which the nurse keeps in the hospital and those in the public health agency. In the latter situation, the record is a family record with individual family members brought into view as they become the focus of attention. The account of the home visit includes observations made, nursing needs identified, action taken, any evidence of results of action taken, goals and plans which the family and the nurse may share, and the nurse's plans for the next visit (including not only the date but purpose and possible preparation of the nurse for that visit). In one writing, the public health nurse incorporates the content found in the hospital situation in the nurse's notes, in the clinical chart, and in the nursing care plan, found usually in a card file.

The advantages the public health nurse enjoys as she shares the nursing record with her co-workers, are found in the unity of the record, its completeness, and its description of the family setting which attunes her to a situation before she enters it. The record she reads reflects a human situation in which evidence is furnished for the judgments and evaluations which have been made. She may feel she can fit into the situation because she is aware of the chain of interaction already begun. On the other hand, the record here described is necessarily a full one and takes time to read. When pressures of many families' nursing needs are great, it sometimes requires considerable self-discipline to read the record before the family visit. Marginal indexes, underlining important points, and particularly periodic summaries at points established by agency policies are excellent ways of streamlining the important task of reading the record in preparation for the visit.

THE PATIENT PORTRAIT AND SUGGESTED APPROACH

In the hospital situation, different but equally pressing urgencies encourage the nurse to omit reading nurse's notes or observations. The acuteness of the hospital situation may make it necessary for the nurse to rely initially upon the nursing care plan to orient her to the patient she is to meet for the first time. Positive responses which have been evoked by particular approaches will be very helpful and should be shared with her in the most expeditious manner possible. Therefore, the nursing care plan, in addition to the nursing diagnosis, nursing care objectives, nursing and medical orders (therapeutic measures), may include a portrait of the patient and ways of working with him which have been helpful. The portrait is an aggregate of all the observations made by nurses who have cared for him, each of whom has perceived him a little differently because each has her own frame of reference.

All nurses must know how to work cooperatively with another human being. However, when nursing needs are to be met by several individuals, whatever briefing can be done as to what has proved to work in general, leads to consistency in approach and to a decreasing demand upon the patient for continual adjustment to changing personnel. In no way is the individual nurse compelled to mimic the approach used by another. She is simply given a clue to some of the many factors that may affect the patient's reaction to her nursing care.

The following are examples of patient portraits and approaches, actual summaries from the nurse's notes which appear on the nursing care plan:

Portrait. Mr. P calls himself "an old New England Yankee from way back." Before his hospitalization, he was considering moving to the apartment of an unmarried sister. While he was living alone, an older, retired brother had been giving him some financial help. He reports that his children do not come to see him much anymore, though one son-in-law has urged him to live with his family at a nearby rural village. Mr. P. takes five to six glasses of an alcoholic beverage every day to keep him going. His work has always been hard physical labor.
Approach. Mr. P. accepts innovations in care if he is first given the opportunity to tell what he tried and what he found successful. He has been ingenious in handling a persistent diarrhea and appreciates commendation for being able to remain independent so long.

Portrait. Mrs. C., a gentle, soft-spoken woman, is the oldest of seven children in an Italian family, having started to work at 16 to help support the family. She married at 22. She and her husband had resented the first pregnancy but loved the baby dearly when he arrived. She feels her present illness is punishment for her early resentment. She is ambitious, teachable, and eager to make a good home for her husband and child.

Approach. Getting Mrs. C. to talk about her baby helps her, in turn, to talk about herself. She responds when sufficient time is spent in giving her nursing care in a deliberate, unhurried manner.

Portrait. Mary S. has a metallic, too-ready laugh. She talks rapidly in a rather high-pitched voice. She suddenly broke her engagement one month ago, certain she had cancer. The marriage was to have been in six months. She says she has been unable to control her emotions, and has been trying to get the most out of everything before she dies. In her quieter moments, she refers to family arguments which have occurred only recently.

Approach. When Mary S. is encouraged to recognize how fear affects emotional control, she is able to express her concern over the rift with her family. Whatever helps her to gain self-understanding seems to bring her nearer to working with what is, to her, the real problem just now—her break with her family.

Some readers may justifiably regard the *Approach* as a nursing measure or nursing action concerned with giving supportive nursing care and therefore to be placed in the nursing care plan in equal rank with specific nursing activities (for example, giving medications, therapeutic diets, teaching crutch-walking, turning each hour, etc.). If this view is taken, the *Approach* is written in a similar, directed style: "give nursing care in a deliberate, unhurried manner," "commend him for remaining independent so long." There may be a danger here in so ordering the nurse's action that she is not free to be herself. She may not be a deliberate, unhurried person. What is more to the point, such a manner might be most inappropriate in the particular situation she and the patient may find themselves. It is best to view the *Approach* as a general guide to patterning the nurse's actions with the patient in question.

Identifying Data

On the nursing care plan, identifying data should be kept at a minimum in order to avoid unnecessary duplication and to avoid the human tendency to short-cut reading the complete record. Name, age, religion, occupation, medical diagnosis, surgical procedure(s) performed, attending physician—these are probably the most immediately useful identifying information. One of the resources the nurse will use early to amplify her own observation and direct communication with the patient will be the medical history found in the clinical chart.

Nurse's Orders or Nursing Measures to Be Taken

On the nursing care plan, nursing care activities are usually grouped as those concerned with 1) giving medications and treatments, special diets, obtaining specimens, and the traditionally transcribed physician's orders and 2) general nursing measures pertaining to personal hygiene or preventive care, instruction, observation, and interpersonal relations. Tremendous advances must be made in the teaching of patients and families. If the patient's needs require predominantly reeducative nursing care, thought must be given to what teaching operation is needed—instruction, interpretation, clarification, giving security, unifying knowledge already possessed with his group culture. Many nurses have not had the opportunity to develop teaching skills. A well-developed in-service workshop on the teaching process, including methods and materials, would help nurses feel much more secure in teaching patients and families.

It must be remembered that a nursing measure may lend itself to the attainment of several nursing care objectives. It may also fall into several categories of nursing care. For example, a preventive measure may also be supportive as well as reeducative. If the nurse's perception of the patient is that of a whole person, then the care she gives will be comprehensive and will be perceived by the patient as helpful in meeting his needs. The written plan is the product of a process which the nurse, patient, or family must have experienced, or no change in the quality of the nursing care she administers can be expected.

NURSE'S ORDERS AS A LEGAL RECORD

In many situations, it has been possible to provide, by way of the nursing care plan, a legal record of medications given, with date and hour and initials of the nurse giving the drug. In the case of drugs given when needed (p.r.n.), these were also charted on the nursing care plan with date, hour, and first initial and surname of the nurse. When such recording is made possible, nurse's notes or observation records need not contain statements of drugs, dosage, route, hour given, and by whom. Such verbatim copy work completely precludes any possibility of the nurse using the observation sheet as a tool for collecting data to determine nursing needs and to evaluate the patient's progress. A legal record is necessary to show that "due care" has been given, but check spaces on the nursing care plan could easily serve this purpose.

Whatever part of the nursing care plan is to serve as a legal record must be kept in ink. Those entries which state the nursing diagnosis, nursing care objectives, and nursing measures should be in pencil. Working with pencil reinforces the idea that the plan is a dynamic, flexible one, the product of continuing reassessment, goal-setting, and decisions for action.

Evaluation of Patient's Progress

There seems to be a general agreement that the nursing care plan should include an evaluation of the patient's progress towards the desired goals. Since the evidence to be used in the evaluation of his progress can only be found in his behavior, there must be a careful description of that behavior. That portion of the clinical chart called "Nurse's Notes," or better still, "Observation of Patient's Behavior," seems more appropriate than the nursing care plan for the description of behavior, whether nursing needs are being identified or progress is being evaluated. The record form could provide three vertical columns designated as: Description of Behavior, Nursing Needs, Progress Towards Goals. The observation sheet truly becomes the source of information as to the patient's strengths and weaknesses and his condition of dis-ease. Here is found the material from which a nursing diagnosis is initially made and is later revised. Here is found in the report of the patient's progress some idea as to the effectiveness of a nursing approach or a nursing action. Description of the patient's behavior provides such essential data, it seems to deserve ample space and considerable emphasis. On the other hand, the nursing care plan is a working tool which can, at any point in time, be substantiated by the data found in the "Observation of the Patient's Behavior."

The Teaching Plan

Occasionally a detailed plan for the instruction of a patient and family members needs to be shared to provide continuity. Content, methods and materials used, who is instructed and how often, whether there have been return demonstrations, whether there will be continued supervision in the home should be recorded in a teaching plan. Not all patients will require a teaching plan, but when one is necessary, it is attached as an addendum to the nursing care plan.

The Form Used for the Nursing Care Plan

Various forms for the nursing care plan have been developed. Some are modifications of the former nurse's order sheet, and others use the Kardex file card, in which case both sides of the card are used. Since the nursing care plan is a working tool, the form should be developed, revised, and perfected by those who use it. The best forms have been worked out by the nursing staff and are therefore unique to various institutions or units within the institution. Where organized group nursing or authentic nursing teams exist, the nursing care plan is recognized as essential, and initiative and creativeness have been demonstrated in devising an effective tool.

The nursing care plan has often been developed by students as a kind of intellectual discipline followed through to the satisfaction of the instructor. The nursing care plan has been shared by the instructor and student, but not with co-workers. It has resided in the instructor's or student's desk drawer or possibly in the student's corner at the head nurse's station. There has been little evidence of its being shaped, changed, or redesigned by all those involved in helping the patient and family attain the objectives of his nursing care. The plan has truly not been the product of the on-going human process of planning. Too often, the young nurse practitioner refers to the nursing care plan as something she wrote when she was a student.

Today, the existence of nursing care plans for each patient is a criterion used in the appraisal of agencies for reimbursements from Medicare and Medicaid programs. There is always the danger that the existence of a form for a nursing care plan may gain the stamp of approval, rather than the presence of the process which creates the form. Once again, the comprehension of the nurse determines the comprehensiveness of the nursing care. How was the form developed? Has it been modified and revised to make it more useful? Is there available a record of the data on which the plan is based? Is time provided and used for planning? The answers to such questions give greater assurance of comprehensive nursing care than does the form of a nursing care plan.

The Nursing Care Study

The nursing care study probably began as a case study which followed an outline covering medical diagnosis, etiology, signs and symptoms, course of the disease, therapy, and prognosis. Nursing care was mentioned in a final brief paragraph stating whatever modifications were required to fit the needs of the individual patient. A case study was usually required of the student in each clinical service. In time, more emphasis was placed upon nursing care, and the final paragraph was greatly expanded.

Today the nursing care study is beginning to have a new meaning. It is being recognized as a professional tool which can be used to evaluate the response of groups of patients to specific nursing measures. Such a study would be feasible and not unreasonable to expect of nursing practitioners who had available nursing care plans and observation of behavior records such as those described in this chapter. It could be a very exciting experience for staff nurses to compare, for example, the responses of patients A, B, and C—all housewives between the ages of 30 and 40 with multiple sclerosis—to specific nursing approaches and nursing measures used over a given period of time. The nursing care study carried out in a practice situation assumes the proportions of preresearch investigation and can become a stepping stone to the measurement of effectiveness of nursing care.

Summary

The nursing care plan contains the most essential identifying data, the nursing diagnoses, the immediate and long-term nursing objectives, the portrait of the patient, and nursing measures or actions related to supportive, remedial, reeducative, and preventive nursing care. General approach to the patient may be described briefly. The evaluation of the patient's progress may be included in the nursing care plan, but this is probably more useful as part of the ongoing description of the patient's behavior recorded elsewhere. A teaching plan which incorporates special plans for discharge may be necessary for some patients, and this is attached to the nursing care plan.

The nursing care plan should be shared by all who participate in the care of the patient and should therefore be accessible and easily available to them. It in no way replaces the recording of observations and communications with the patient and the identification of nursing needs.

8

Implementing the Nursing Care Plan

To carry out a plan involves the selection and use of resources, both human and material, which will best serve to accomplish the established objectives. Material resources which contribute to meeting health goals are physical and economic in nature. For example, light, heat, water, food, means of transportation, shelter or housing, finances, and equipment are necessary to carry out any plan of continuous, extended, and comprehensive nursing care. Human resources lie not only within the nurse and the patient, but within all the human groups to which each relates.

Human Resources

In earlier chapters, the resources of the patient, his family, and the nurses were explored in terms of planning nursing care. An estimate was made of the patient's health knowledge and his use of it, his motivation, his attitudes, his compensatory and control mechanisms, the use he had made of past experiences, his interpersonal relationships, and how he related his health status to other goals. The nurse took stock of her own past experiences, recognizing differences and similarities in them and the present situation. She examined her attitudes and feelings and considered her skills in terms of what would be required.

Within the patient's immediate social setting are many resources, particularly his family, friends, and other patients who share his illness experience with him. The family's resources may be economic, or they may be related to other experiences with illness, interpersonal relationships, management, and problem-solving skills. Other patients have had or are having illness experiences. If these can be used by the patient or the nurse, they provide a very real resource. The resources of the nurse (her own skills and experiences) can be extended by other nurses who work with her in providing the patient with comprehensive nursing care. These are complemented by the skills of other health workers. Thus, the range of resources is a wide and varied one. The selection and use of human resources will be the focal point of this chapter.

The Process of Referral

Selection of resources must be based upon an understanding of the extent and depth of the needs to be met. It may seem relatively simple to categorize man's needs as physical, social, emotional, and spiritual, then to match these needs with those resources best able to fill the gaps. However, as the comprehension of the nature of man grows, and we recognize him as a whole being with an inner compulsion to preserve that wholeness, the matching of needs and resources becomes more complex.

One of the significant outcomes of the ability to perceive human behavior as an expression of interrelated needs is the increase in the overlapping functions of the helping professions. There are marginal areas in which teacher and nurse, nurse and physician, social worker and nurse, nutritionist and nurse work interchangeably, and the preparation of either professional is adequate to perform like functions. For example, both the nurse and social worker are prepared to give supportive care, both use the interview to assess needs within the patient and family group and to define problems. Both are concerned with the inter- and intrapersonal relationships of the patient and his family. Both make use of their ability to work with the patient. The physician and the nurse are both schooled in administering therapeutic measures to relieve functional and organic disorders. Both teacher and nurse counsel, instruct, and help the individual preserve his cultural identity. The acceptance of similarities in the helping professions has made possible an integrative approach to human problems.

DISTINCTIVE SKILLS FOUND
WITHIN EACH HEALTH PROFESSION

Each profession has a focus unique to itself because of its origins and its philosophy. For example, social work has its roots in the Judeo-Christian concern for people who have unusual difficulty in functioning as social and spiritual beings, and in the recognition of the right of self-determination without infringing on the rights of others. The social worker applies the principles of self-determination by helping the individual define his own problem. Every effort is made to see the problem as the patient and the family see it. The social worker uses his knowledge of the psychology of adjustment to increase the client's self-understanding and to help him make decisions which will resolve problems of adjustment to his life-situation. If these objectives are achieved, it is often the social worker who has made it possible for the client-patient to effectively use health services and to carry out a therapeutic regime.

In contrast, the physician belongs to a profession associated with healing. To restore to health is to make whole that individual who, for the time being, is dependent or less than whole. Self-determination and decision-making is not always possible when treatment is necessary to make one whole. The physician decides that treatment must be instituted. Not only the dependency of the ill individual, but the uncommon knowledge which the physician possesses, has created a deeply-rooted belief in the doctor's curative ability.

The nurse belongs to a profession rooted in the art of nurture. To nurture is to nourish, to protect, to provide an environment in which it is possible to grow and to flourish. To protect from harm and to care for means supplying those things and performing those acts which the patient cannot provide and do for himself.

The profession of the ministry is established on the belief in man's relationship to a divine purpose, to an ultimate source of goodness, to an infinite fount of life—in short, to God as He is revealed to man. The minister, whether rabbi, clergyman, or priest, is especially prepared to help the individual meet this need to feel a part of a greater whole, to find new meaning in his life experiences because he can relate himself to a goodness greater than that which lies within him.

An understanding, then, of the depth as well as the range of needs of the patient and his family helps the nurse to recognize when and what other resources must be used. To some extent she can help the patient and family meet their spiritual needs. Kind and loving care, sensitive response in those moments when the patient questions why ill fortune has befallen him or when the patient or his family want to talk about or to a supreme being, the expression of her own attitudes toward suffering, old age, death, bereavement, or birth—these are concrete ways of meeting spiritual needs. Too often, the nurse perceives meeting spiritual needs in terms of honoring a dietary regulation or respecting special requests for religious ceremonies at time of birth or terminal illness. Without some mode of expressing her own spiritual self, her knowledge of the practices and observances of various religious denominations makes it possible for her to act only as a facilitator, not as a resource for the patient and family.

However, there are levels of spiritual need which the nurse is not prepared to meet, and referral to a spiritual advisor is indicated. She then helps the patient seek the rabbi or clergyman and makes it possible within the hospital, home, or nursing home, for the patient to make the fullest use of spiritual aid. Likewise, there are levels of medical and social need which she is not prepared to meet. Referral to physician and social worker then becomes her responsibility.

WHO IS INVOLVED IN SELECTING RESOURCES?

Those who are to use the resource must be involved in the selection of the resource. Ideally, the choice is made by the patient and family, always based upon an assessment of the need and upon adequate information as to what the resource is able to provide. The nurse may find the patient's and family's perception of the resource is limited by lack of information, by previous experience, or by the public image of the resource person. Do the patient and his family associate the social worker with financial inadequacy? Perhaps the use of social services always implies inadequacies in family relationships, and consequently this resource is a threat to family integrity. Does the family always associate the physician with illness and health emergencies? Is the clergyman viewed as the forerunner of death, the last resort in terminal illness? Often the nurse's task is to help another change his view of what a resource can offer. She often does this by illustration or by helping the patient and family explore the resource before using it fully. When the need engulfs them and robs them of the ability to make decisions, the nurse must give the patient and his family very specific information about the resource, introduce each to the other, even help them select the basic information to be shared.

Within the hospital setting, the nurse often relates the patient to the community resource through the medical social worker. This agent knows the setting within which the resource person works, the criteria for eligibility, the scope and limitations of the services the agency's program provides, the established fees for services. Since patients often do not direct questions to those best qualified to answer them, but to those with whom they have the most personal contact, the nurse in the hospital should be familiar with the basic information about community services. Some hospitals make available to the staff in nursing units a community directory of health, social, and welfare agencies. This practice helps to develop the concept of the hospital as a part of the community and a link in a chain of continuing care.

The public health nurse in the home and community setting must have detailed information about community agencies. Because her contact with them is direct, she is able either to refer the patient and family directly to the resource or to aid them in selection of the resource.

SELECTING INFORMATION TO BE SHARED

The exchange of information is a crucial element in the process of referral. The purpose of the referral usually indicates what information is pertinent. In nurse-to-nurse referral, the purpose is usually related to extending some aspect of nursing care; for example, helping a patient adjust to a new prosthesis, to accept and follow a therapeutic diet, to care for a new baby, or helping a family member give basic nursing care to the patient in the home. In each instance, pertinent information would include what help has been given by the nurse initiating the referral, what has been the response of the patient and the progress he has made, what methods and approaches have been helpful, how much is the patient able to do for himself, and what might be the next steps. The referring nurse shares the present nursing care objectives so that ongoing nursing care is goal-directed.

Since nursing care is always correlated with medical care, a nurse referral must include information concerning medical supervision. Often physician-to-physician and nurse-to-nurse referrals occur simultaneously. In this case, the physician selects and shares pertinent information with his colleague, but he must remember that the nurse implements those aspects of the medical care plan that affect the functions of the whole patient—his activity, rest, and healing processes. What does the physician mean by "bed rest," "limited activities," "application of heat," and other general phrases?

When the purpose of referral originates primarily from other than health needs, the nurse again must select pertinent information. Often she is reluctant to share because she is dealing with personal information entrusted to her by the patient and family. Preferably, she makes it possible for them to share directly such information by helping them recognize what would be useful to the resource person or by helping them become uncomfortable with the latter. Some social workers feel the information a client shares directly is most significant, since the sharing is part of the process of relating, and relating is a part of therapy. Therefore, the social worker may wish only identifying data from the referring person or agency.

There are times when patients and families need to have others speak for them. Statements describing observable behavior reduce the danger of prejudicing another or setting a stage. However, an interpretation of behavior reveals something of the patient's relationship to the referring person and may be valuable in appraising his past experience. When the nurse includes an interpretation of behavior she needs to give some basis for her interpretation. For example, "I find Mrs. A. feels very apprehensive about possible emergencies which could arise in the care of her husband's tracheotomy tube. She has given her husband care in the hospital but has asked repeatedly, 'What do I do if he chokes up?' "

As the referring person, the nurse must often serve as a sounding-board, not only for the patient and family but for those to whom they have been referred. Frequently agency workers call upon the nurse to supplement their experiences with the client by sharing her own. Comparison of responses helps the worker to reexamine his approach, to see the client in other situations, and perhaps to gain some self-insight. Case conferences which include the referring person have proved extremely helpful in guaranteeing the effectiveness of the referral.

EVALUATION OF THE OUTCOME

A benefit of the continuing contact between the referring person and the resource is an opportunity for an evaluation of the act of referral. Was the original purpose of the referral achieved? Did the patient and family receive nursing care as long as needed, as long as they felt they needed it? Was the orientation of the patient and his family to the resource such that they were able to make use of it? Was sufficient information supplied concerning the care the patient and family had been receiving? Was the purpose of referral justifiable? Was referral made too soon, too late? Was referral used as a means of avoidance or escape? Was the nurse so personally involved she could not relinquish the patient when his needs were no longer nursing needs? Evaluation is essential, not only to improve the nurse's judgment in selecting a resource, but also to give her the satisfaction of knowing the outcome of the referral. She needs to feel that she has been able to extend herself as a helping person and that she can work constructively with other helping people.

One aspect of the follow-through which complete evaluation requires has often been neglected. This is the effort to obtain from the person or persons referred an expression of what referral meant to them. What was their experience in terms of adjustment, of awareness of their role, of further assistance in becoming independent? Not all patient and families may be able to share their feelings, but those who can will make quite clear their feelings of sustained support or of continuous buffeting from pillar to post.

The process of referral which may occur in the use of resources may be summarized as one in which 1) the need is matched with the resource best able to meet the need, and 2) the patient is helped to recognize the need, to know the resource and the kind of help it offers, to accept and subsequently seek the resource, and to use it effectively. The helping act includes introducing the patient to the resource, giving pertinent information to both the patient and the receiving agent, and following through and evaluating the results of the referral. To insure continuity of care there must be continuous interchange, continuous reassessment of the need, and evaluation of the extent to which it is being met. Referral is an ongoing process in which the patient and family are actively involved and, if possible, initiate the process.

THE REFERRAL FORM

Whatever form is developed to serve as a written record of referral, it must provide the requisites of purposeful and satisfying interchange between sender and receiver. Therefore, it must contain:

1. Full identifying data.
2. Accurate and full instructions as to how to contact the individual being referred.
3. Pertinent and specific information as to the care given and to be extended, anticipated needs, and plans for meeting them. Care refers to that given by the physician, nurse, social worker, physical therapist, nutritionist, and others, i.e., by all health workers who have been involved. Details of care such as limited activities, bed rest, diet, etc. must be described specifically.
4. Provision for continuing reports from those receiving the patient to those referring him, and vice versa.

The written referral should become a permanent part of the patient's record in both the sending and receiving agency.

PART III

Providing for Nursing Care

9

Groups Who Work Together

In recent years, the group and its behavior has been a major concern, even the focus of investigative study. Man has always lived in a social setting in which he has achieved self-identity through his group experiences. With urban living and the growing population, these experiences have increased and he moves in and out of a maze of group associations.

The Nature of a Group

Sociologists designate the family as the prototype of the true group. The family has a definite membership. Each member is expected to play a certain role acceptable to him and recognized by other members as appropriate. The members of the family group have common goals. Sometimes these goals cannot be verbally expressed by a family member, but they nevertheless serve to mobilize the group as a unit in times of crisis and decision-making. The group member has individual goals which may be compatible with family goals. If not, he is able to lay them aside, modify them, or postpone their attainment when their pursuit would interfere with the success of the group. The family member has a strong feeling of belongingness. "We" often replaces "I," and the individual truly identifies with the family group. This feeling of belonging supersedes the individual's identification with an ethnic or ethical group. To the degree a family possesses the four characteristics—a sense of belonging, common goals, definite membership, accepted and recognized member roles—it is a group, an entity with an identity of its own.

Early in life, the individual moves into other groups such as the play group, school group, the innumerable peer groups of the adolescent, the church group, the fraternity or lodge, and so on. To the extent any one of these secondary groups takes on the described characteristics of the primary or family group, that group may become a primary group and a kind of substitute family for the individual. This substitution occurs more and more often when the family becomes increasingly ineffective as a true group. On the other hand, the individual may find no group able to substitute for the family group, and, even though he moves in and out of a myriad of groups, he may never achieve a feeling of belonging, a feeling of some unity by which he can find himself.

Two characteristics of today's society contribute to the inability of groups to provide for the individual an opportunity for self-identification. The mobility of the population, in general, prevents any kind of permanency or definition of membership in a group. Without some degree of permanency, roles cannot be defined or accepted. The second characteristic is a lack of direction or purpose. Mobility and lack of direction, coupled with man's need for belonging, have resulted in much emphasis upon togetherness and group activity. Togetherness without direction or purpose has resulted in fragmented group experience and the tragic feeling of loneliness and anonymity in the midst of groups.

Group Tasks and the Roles of Group Members

A true group has two tasks—that of attaining its goals (this amounts to getting its work done) and that of maintaining its wholeness or integrity as a group. The accomplishment of these two tasks helps a group to remain whole, to remain sound and healthy, and to grow in productiveness. One task may take precedence over the other at a given point in time, but both are always present as a means of cementing the group. If a priority must be set, then the task of keeping the group whole by meeting the needs of individual members must be undertaken first. The group can never be considered of greater importance than the individual within the group.

Each individual within the true group assumes a role acceptable to him and the group. The role he assumes is not assigned to him but grows out of the way he relates to others, his commitment to the goals of the group, the degree of self-realization he possesses, how he perceives himself, and what is expected of him by the group. These factors determine whether his role will be directed more to the group-task or to group-maintenance. If task-directed, he may be described as the one in the group who gives and seeks information, who clarifies, summarizes, records, and keeps order. If his role is more concerned with maintaining the group's wholeness, he may be found keeping the peace, helping group members express themselves, and harmonizing conflicts.

Group-member roles may be also established by the culture of the society within which the group exists. The professional roles of physician, social worker, teacher, and lawyer, have been identified not only by the profession but by society. Likewise, the roles of leader, observer, and recorder have been quite carefully described by groups. In the family group, certain members have had roles ascribed to them because of their position in the group. For example, the father has been described as the wage earner, the mother as the homemaker, the eldest son as the standardsetter, the mother-in-law as obstacle-maker or opposer. Roles change and are never static, but they must always be concerned with one or both of the group tasks.

Leadership Within a Group

As the group moves into getting its work done, a kind of sorting-out takes place which leads to the development of levels or strata within the group. Individual experience, educational preparation, talent or intellectual ability, the seniority which time may have given an individual— these and other factors lead to establishing a position or status. Responsibility and authority are delegated with respect to the group task. Organization has resulted from the sorting, classifying, and arranging of levels or strata.

Much has been written about the position of the group leader. Is leadership located in one individual or does it reside in the group itself? Is leadership fixed or always emerging and moving? Often an individual has been designated as group leader when the real leadership lies in those who named him leader. Very probably, leadership grows out of commitment to the values of the group. Belief in something and willingness to work hard for it is essential to leadership whether it reside in an individual or in a group. John Gardner[1] has said, "Neither intellect nor talent can be the key to leadership positions. The additional requirement is commitment to the highest values of that society."

Leadership behavior has been described as authoritatian, laissez-fair, or democratic. Authoritarian leadership exerts authority because of position in the group. The effectiveness of that leadership will depend largely upon the process by which the position was created (the involvement of the group in sorting, classifying, organizing, defining positions). Laissez-fair leadership is often found in groups who have not defined their goals, or in groups where individual member goals are not compatible with those of the group. In order to keep some semblance of group wholeness, the group avoids seeking direction and permits itself to be buffeted about by the individual wills. Democratic leadership is leadership of the group by the group, for what it holds most dear—the realization of individual and group potentials to be and do their best as they see it.

It is imperative to recognize that choice of leadership lies with the group. The leader represents what the group consciously or unconsciously ascribes to and holds dear. Leadership behavior will depend upon the amount of group involvement in defining goals and values and upon the amount of commitment to those goals and values.

Desirable change implies two things: an awareness of some worthwhile end or goal to be attained, and an awareness that change is needed to reach that goal. Setting up goals involves conscious focus upon some desired end, a reaching out for some distant point. What is hoped for depends upon values. Any group in setting goals moves through a period in which individual values are shared, compared, and contrasted. The extent to which group members are able to talk out what they believe in, what their individual hopes and desires are, determines to a large degree the clarity of group goals. This period in which a group philosophy or system of beliefs evolves provides a kind of centripetal force which leads to the formation of a group identity, the core of a true group. The individual who is action- or present-oriented often finds this period very frustrating. He may take a position aloof from the group or even leave it completely.

As goals are defined, what is required to meet those goals becomes apparent. Rarely are these two steps taken in a sequential order.[2] Individuals within a group vary in their approach. Some will be more concerned with defining needs. Others will be quite clear as to goals but unsure of what is needed to reach those goals. Individual approaches complement each other so that recognized goals and recognized needs provide the motivation for the group.

Motivation leads to action which involves joint planning, decision making, and delegation of authority and responsibility for specific tasks. Planning engages group members in exploring how a need could be supplied, what could be done, and what consequences might be expected. Resources are examined in terms of people, materials, and finances. Actions which other groups have taken and the outcomes of those actions are often examined. The group engages in gathering information, selecting information that is pertinent to the goals and to their diagnosis of needs to be met, and arranging the information into some design of action. Many kinds of decisions are made. Which goal is most immediate? What needs must first be met? What action promises the greatest measure of success? Which action is most feasible in terms of resources available? Is there any way in which an action could be put to test before the group finally decides to take that action?

Decisions must be carried out. During the process described in preceding paragraphs, leadership within the group has emerged. Skill or expertise is recognized in the individual member with respect to his use of the information he possesses, his preparation for and experience in some given area. When authority is recognized, responsibility is given to that individual by the group. He becomes the group leader with respect to the group task. Another kind of leadership is needed, that of keeping the group whole. This leadership, too, emerges from the group, and an individual may excel in this kind of expertise. In a true group, responsibility for group action and for group integrity lies, in the final analysis, within the group itself.

Such responsibility involves the evaluation of not only the product

but the process of group action. The individual within the group tends
to focus upon the product or the process because of the nature of the
role he has assumed. Sometimes he is recognized by the group as the
one most sensitive to group process and is asked to help the group look
at what is happening and what contributes to the group's wholeness. A
group as a whole seems frequently to be more capable of evaluating the
outcome of its actions, *the product,* than appraising the dynamics of
the interrelationships of group members, *its process.* Therefore, a group
may use a group member as an observer of process. However, the
ultimate desire of a true group is to have every member engaged in
evaluation of both process and product.

Effecting Change Within a Group

In the administration of comprehensive nursing care, the nurse
associates with many groups. These groups include the family group,
co-worker groups often called the "nursing team" or "health team,"
and various kinds of community groups. The nurse also has associations
with professional organizations. Often these are called groups, but they
lack some of the characteristics of the true group which have been
previously described. However, when the purpose of the nurse's
association with a professional organization is to effect the administration of comprehensive nursing care, then she regards it as potentially a
true group which may be instrumental in bringing about change. Her
success depends upon her understanding of group behavior and her
ability to help the group bring about the change necessary to administer
comprehensive nursing care. She is concerned with the group goal and
with group action. She is engaged in bringing about group cooperation,
an essential element of administration.

Lippit[3] has described three phases of planned change which create a
kind of cyclic motion moving from unfreezing the present state to a
new level and finally to stabilizing group life at a new level. Abstract as
this description of planned change may seem, the phases can be clearly
identified in group life as change-agents are introduced.

As the nurse enters a group, her first task is that of assessing or appraising forces within individuals and within the group which operate for or against change. Ruth Freeman[4] points out dissatisfaction with what one is doing as one of the major forces contributing to change. Relating the individual's goals to group goals, whether they may be improving a patient's care, getting more information, or increasing one's status, will help an individual accept change. He loses nothing and gains much as he participates in effecting change.

Often a satisfying relationship with the nurse herself, or some other group member, can serve to make an individual responsive to change. Again, an individual's personal frame of reference is always in the process of change. If more could be known about changes in the foreground of the individual's field, the nurse as a change-agent could capitalize upon changes already taking place.

Not only in individuals, but in groups, organizations, and communities, there are forces favorable to change. Groups which recognize an obstacle to a common goal and whose members have had success in doing something together and feel that new skills have been acquired have developed tremendous momentum for change. If members of the group have a good relationship with the nurse who enters the group as the change-agent, then these forces can be used to full advantage.

In an organization, the desire to produce, to preserve identity, or establish leadership, or the dissatisfaction with returns from efforts put forth create a setting favorable for changes. Large organizations as well as communities have small internal groups where conflict creates unrest and where change is already taking place. The very dynamics of groups in contact with each other means that changing forces are always present as new groups appear, old groups are replaced or assimilated, and the cycle of invasion and succession continues. At the same time, the nurse recognizes in the individual a reluctance to admit a need for change, a feeling of awkwardness and a fear of failure when something new is to be tried. Change means losing some current satisfaction, and perhaps the nurse encounters most often the individual's inability to fix his attention on some end and to define the means to that end.

As she enters a co-worker group, she often encounters unawareness of interpersonal relationships, resistance to self-appraisal, and the absence of any group criteria for self-evaluation. As she moves into larger groups, organizations, and communities, she finds that change threatens productivity and the status quo of posts of authority and status. Often the large group has developed no mechanisms for making decisions. Perhaps the greatest obstacle in the large group is the low degree of responsibility for general welfare which results from the absence of real emotional involvement with each other.

The Nurse and the Family Group

Certain factors are unique to the family group. The nurse is never a permanent member of this group; she is a kind of adjunct member or a consultant to the group and can never relate to family members as a peer. Her objectives for the family are often not in agreement with the family's own goals. She has no part in the group's previous experiences and has not moved through the phases of development in family living. Therefore, common ground must be discovered. Again, she alone has knowledge of group process. She cannot, as in other groups with whom she works, expect members of the family group to use consciously the principles of involvement, joint planning, permissiveness, contrast, and feedback which insure effective group work.

In the first phase of effecting change, the nurse makes herself available to the family and increases their awareness of the kinds of help she can give them. She recognizes a family member who is a potential change-agent and relates to that individual. She tries to help the family identify its goals, the obstacles to meeting those goals, the successes it has had, the resources it has used or failed to use, or the unavailable resources. In short, this phase is a period of assessment, orientation, and diagnosis.

Out of this period develops either a redefinition of long-term goals which are mutually acceptable to the nurse and family or the selection of a goal which can be readily attained. Some measure of success motivates the family to undertake further change. The nurse supplies knowledge in health matters, informs the family of resources related to their needs, and she may even serve as a liaison between the family and the church, school, hospital clinic, or community agency.

Finally, once change is effected, the nurse reinforces those factors in the family group which will help sustain and perpetuate the change.

She helps the family evaluate itself, compare the present with the past, and perceive that further change will take place so that ongoing progress becomes acceptable. In every way possible, she nourishes and protects the growing areas in family life.

The Nurse and the Nurse-Practitioner Group

In effecting change in the nurse-practitioner group, the nurse finds herself in a very different situation from that in the family group. In the former, she is a group member, sharing common goals and experiences with nurse-practitioners who are concerned with patient welfare. The nurse-practitioner group here includes only those licensed to provide nursing care and excludes the many individuals now assigned to technical procedures and activities.

In the period of assessing the nurse-practitioner group, the nurse has to consider the different educational orientation of group members. In spite of the professed commitment of educational programs to prepare nurse-practitioners who give patient-centered care, one must admit that many learning experiences still lead her to focus upon tasks to be done, technical devices to operate or to monitor, and routines to follow. Awareness of the different perceptions of the act of nursing helps the nurse accept the members of the nursing group. She understands the meaning of work to the individual and how each member perceives her role. Again, the nurse, if she is to be a change-agent, becomes conscious of the range of skills in a nurse-practitioner group. This assessment of nursing resources in the group gives her insight to where successes and personal satisfactions lie and where professional growth is taking place.

The position of the individual nurse-practitioner in the hierarchy of the nurse-practitioner group must be considered. Unfortunately, for many individuals, progression up the ladder is synonymous with success. The individual's comprehension of the institutional or agency framework in which she works is very limited; she is sensitive to promotion upward, and she is often uninformed as to the total context of the organization in which she works and unaware of horizontal or staff relationships. The nurse team or group as a small operational unit is still a very new concept. In insitutions where it has been recognized, it has frequently not attained sufficient cohesiveness to become a real entity or to develop characteristics of a true group. Too often, the group has been set up as a team to divide tasks to be performed, to enhance further the status acquired by educational preparation and not by proved competence in giving excellent nursing care. This so-called group has not developed the characteristics of the true group; there is no feeling of belonging together growing out of common goals, accepted roles, and a definite membership.

The nurse, as a change-agent in the nurse-practitioner group, moves through the same three phases of effecting change which were described with the family group. She relates to the individual nurse as an accepting, understanding person. She learns to know her satisfactions, her frustrations, and her professional background. She makes it acceptable to question, to explore, and even to complain. Often there is an immediate opportunity to establish herself as the helping person, the person who can clarify elements in the situation or serve as a liaison with resource people of whom the individual may be unaware or whom she is reluctant to approach.

Always the nurse watches and listens for an awareness of patients' problems. With the group, she helps them identify common problems, establish goals, and select action necessary to reach those goals. Whenever possible, she reminds the group of the common goal of excellent nursing care to patients and families. She explores with the group its criteria for excellent nursing care. Perhaps her greatest advantage in the nursing group is the opportunity to demonstrate optimum quality of nursing care. Often setting a model which provides evidence of the effectiveness of a measure or action different from the customary one serves as a powerful instrument to bring about change. Because the nurse has much in common with other members of the group, the kind of direct nursing care to patients she demonstrates is perhaps her most eloquent means of communication in motivating others to improve the quality of nursing care.

Other methods the nurse may use are manifold. Nursing care conferences held by the group offer tremendous possibilities for the development of a relatively permanent, stable group. The daily conference is considered to be the core of the team pattern of patient care. In the conference some phase of the nursing process is examined, and the group members begin to see themselves as valued, contributing members, each an integral part of the group. Leadership within the group becomes evident during the conference. It is important to have a designated leader, selected by virtue of experience, preparation, and demonstrated expertise in giving nursing care. This delegation of leadership responsibility affords the group security and continuity but in no way negates the leadership that grows out of the dynamics of the conference. The development of nursing care plans is another excellent method of giving the group an experience in which they become more aware of common goals and their interdependence in carrying out and evaluating the outcomes of nursing actions.

Studies of aspects of patient care serve to develop a group's self-awareness as well as its evaluative skills. Esther Lucille Brown's[5] suggestions as to what might be studied have actually been carried out by some nursing groups as exploratory, investigative studies. What behavior of staff do patients find annoying? What patient behavior determines the nurses' descriptions of "problem patient," "uncooperative," "demanding," or "hostile?" How do nurses assess health counseling needs of patients, and how and when is that counseling given? What physical rearrangements of the ward could be made to facilitate patient socialization? What is the effect of the intercommunication system upon the kinds of nurse-patient communication? What kinds of nursing needs require referral to the community nursing service? Simple studies carried on in a systematic, orderly fashion stimulate deliberate, critical thinking and a search for interrelated cause and effect factors. The staff member will return again and again to the nursing situation to validate her observations, to observe with greater acuity, and to resort to instruments and aids which extend her direct observations. To effect change in the nurse-practitioner group, the nurse as change-agent must continuously help the staff be aware of its purposes and directions and become more sensitive to human behavior, its significance, and its origins.

The Nurse and the Basic Interprofessional Group

Administration of comprehensive nursing care frequently requires the nurse to act as a change-agent in the interprofessional group. To understand the nature of this group requires some knowledge of the characteristics of the professional group from which each member comes. The physician belongs to a group whose expertise in the therapeutic or cure function is undisputed. Because of this unchallenged expertise, it is accepted that he work independently of any institutional or agency hierarchy. He is expected to use a wide range of services provided by other healing professions to extend and reinforce the plan of medical care. He is held in esteem as a member of an ancient, highly respected, and awesome profession, the practice of which requires an intellectually exacting and physically rigorous preparation. Above all, his relationship with the patient is recognized as all-important and is not to be disturbed by any intervening agent.

The social worker comes from a professional group committed to a concern with the individual's life situation, his functioning as a social being. Implicit with this concern is the goal of modifying the behavior or the environment of the client, so that he can obtain maximum benefit from the prescribed therapy. The social worker's educational preparation has predisposed him to look at process rather than product, at the dynamics of a situation rather than the outcome. Because he is skilled in analysis of interaction, he can and does examine his own reactions and responses in a worker-client situation. He is sensitive to the client's response to him and to others and is more concerned with multiple interrelationships than with single relationships.

Because of his professional frame of reference, the social worker is accustomed to taking action when the client is ready. He permits the client to set the pace and to help determine the action to be taken. He is highly knowledgeable in terms of the resources which both he and the client may use. The social worker has been schooled to be highly discriminating as to how information provided by the client is used. Before he shares such information he must be very sure of why and how the information is to be used.

In relating to the social worker in the interprofessional group, the nurse as a change-agent needs to be aware that the very sensitivity to the client which is required of the social worker may cause him to set limits in situations involving other professional workers. The social worker, as a human being, needs some safe areas in which he, not someone else, can establish the order, the pace, and even the nature of events to take place. He needs a kind of vent or means of preserving his own sense of wholeness, his equilibrium. The rigidity and reluctance to share, which nurses find frustrating in the social worker as a co-worker, may become less of a threat if the nurse understands and accepts the professional framework within which the social worker operates.

The third member of the basic interprofessional group is the nurse herself. Today, her so-called professional background is a confused one. As a licensed nurse-practitioner, she may be referred to as a professional nurse or a nurse-technician and her preparation described as professional, technical, or vocational. Great confusion exists as to the objectives of the several patterns of nursing education. Consumer expectations have been relatively slow in changing from primarily physical ministration to the exercise of critical judgment, decision-making with respect to emotional support, counseling, and reeducation, which are so characteristic of professional nursing practice. It seems only reasonable that members of the nursing profession, not the consumers of nursing service, carry the responsibility of clearly delineating the essential characteristics of professional practice.

The nurse belongs to a group whose traditions are rooted in religious and militaristic social systems. The influence of one in its most extreme manifestations is expressed in self-denial, in dedication of self to the relief of the suffering, even in martyrdom. Comfort to those in physical distress and solace to the dying stem from the Judeo-Christian origins of nursing. On the other hand, vertical lines of command with the fragmentation of collective effort which occurs when decisions are made without the involvement of those who are to carry them out—those conditions which have been accepted in nursing for years—have their roots in the militaristic social system. The nurse has been the implementer of orders made by others; she has been the active person in situations where often life itself has been at stake.

In both religious and militaristic social systems, a high degree of individual responsibility and accountability exists. Unfortunately, responsibility has often been assumed without examining what it involves or the authority required to carry out that responsibility. The nurse has often been accountable to more than one unit in the organizational plan. For example, she is responsible to the physician *and* to the director of nursing service, with the latter answerable to the hospital administrator *and* the chief of the medical staff. The nurse may be answerable to the public health director or physician *and* to the school superintendent.

The nurse as well as the physician has had as her primary concern helping people to get well. Dependency needs are predominant in the sick person, so that helping him has meant performing acts for him or directed towards him. Only as the conservation and promotion of health developed as the nurse's concern did she begin to work *with* patients and to help them help themselves. As the person who carries out orders, the nurse has tended to work alone and to be unaware of resources, since resources are sought only when one has some degree of freedom to use them. She has worked within limits established by others. Only with the recognition of the independent functions of the nurse has the use of resources—within herself, in the patient, the family group, and the community—become a part of her preparation. However, whatever limitations have been imposed upon the nurse's functions, it can never be forgotten that she has always had intimate, personal contact with people. She has been in a unique position to recognize the defense lines of an individual, to assess his resources, and to remotivate him.

What can the nurse, whose preparation, cultural background, and assigned position have just been described, do to effect change in the interprofessional group? She can employ three principles proposed by Kenneth Benne[6] in his exposition of the social group as a medium of reeducation: the principles of contrast, involvement and joint planning, and feedback. As she complements the work of other professional health workers, she establishes herself in a role acceptable to them. She brings new insights, helps reorient the group, and "makes it possible for them to perceive and accept alternatives to present practice."[6] Contrast between what is and what might be becomes apparent.

If the nurse takes initiative in involving other members of the interprofessional group in planning the care of the patient, she makes use of the second principle, involvement and planning. This action is often difficult for the nurse to take because it is not a part of the culture of her professional group to take initiative. There are many implications here for the kind of preparation the nurse must have to develop the necessary self-assurance.

When the nurse shares with other members of the interprofessional group the results of jointly planned action, she uses the principle of feedback. Because of her opportunity to observe the patient closely over an extended period of time, she may well provide the evidence needed for the group to evaluate the results of its planning. Specific methods the nurse uses consciously to effect change include making herself available to other professional health workers. She accompanies the physician on visits to the patient to whom they jointly provide care. She makes herself known and available to the physician. Again, she seeks out other group members as consultants or resource persons in the nurse group's conferences. She sets up planned conferences on the ward or in the community agency for the interprofessional group. She organizes information she can give the group about patients and families, and she formulates questions which can be directed to another professional worker whom she can expect to have the answer. She may contact the physician in his office, or telephone him at a time he has designated, with organized information or formulated questions. In short, she uses her group work skills to make it possible for group members to contribute fully and to insure the quality of her own contributions.

The Nurse and Community Groups

The citizen or community group, with which the nurse is often temporarily involved, is less discrete and much more complex in its motivations and goals than any of the groups thus far described. However, it is with this group she often works to effect change in the setting or environment of the individual. She is concerned with those factors in his environment which predispose him to illness or precipitate and perpetuate illness.

In order to act as a change-agent with the community group, the nurse must know a great deal about the community at large. What groups of individuals possess the power to influence others? What groups are in the process of change? Where does leadership lie? What plans for change have already been implemented successfully? In what areas of community life does she find representation from many different groups?

Methods the nurse uses to effect change in the community group are similar to those she has used with other groups; here she must make herself available as a resource person to many groups, involving citizens as volunteer groups. She selects key persons in community groups to whom she interprets nursing services. She keeps groups informed of resources, both individuals and agencies. She invites community groups to conduct self-surveys and community surveys. She continually allies herself as a professional person with groups in which there is a broad community representation.

Summary

An ever-growing understanding of group behavior and increasing skill in helping a group bring about desired change are essential to the administration of comprehensive nursing care. As she assesses group member roles and evaluates group behavior, the nurse becomes deeply involved with the essential task of maintaining group integrity. As she helps a group shake itself free of one state, move to a new level, and stabilize itself at the new level, she is engaged in the other group task of accomplishing a goal. Cooperation, an essential element of administration, is synonymous with effective group interaction. The acquisition of skill in working with groups, then, becomes imperative for the nurse-practitioner.

References

1. Gardner, J. Excellence. New York, Harper and Brothers, 1961.
2. Symonds, P. What Education Has to Learn from Psychology, 3rd ed. New York, Teachers College, Columbia University, 1965.
3. Lippit. R., Watson, J., and Westley, B. The Dynamics of Planned Change: A Comparative Study of Principles and Techniques. New York, Harcourt, Brace & World, Inc., 1958.
4. Freeman, R. Public Health Nursing, 3rd ed. Philadelphia, W.B. Saunders Co., 1963.
5. Brown, E.L. Newer Dimensions of Patient Care. New York, Russell Sage Foundation, 1961, Vol. 1.

6.   Benne, K.D. The Small Group as a Medium of Re-education. Boston
     University Human Relations Center, Research Reports and
     Technical Notes, No. 8.

10

Coordination as an Element of Administration

Cooperation requires coordination, perhaps the most complex element in administration. In the effort to clarify professional nursing practice, care, cure, and coordination have been listed as its three essential components. There have been many reactions to what may be an over-simplified description. However, the concept of coordination cannot be avoided if comprehensive nursing care is to be administered.

If one considers coordination within the human organism, he thinks of the articulation of joints, the harmonious movements of muscle groups, the interrelationships of systems in the body—in short, the smooth working of the human organism as a whole as opposed to the operation of each of its functional parts. The organism's unified activity depends not on the parts alone but on how they relate to one another. Reciprocal relationships found in the origin and insertion of muscles or in the release of hormones within the body create an interdependence which makes it possible for the human organism to operate as a whole.

If one's focus shifts to the institution or agency within which a group or groups work as a whole, one finds an interlocking of effort, a structuring of relationships which are the outcomes of the act of coordination. Mary Follett[1] states that every organization has a form or structure, and what the organization does, its unified activity, depends not on the constituent elements alone but on how these constituents are related one to another.

The nurse who administers comprehensive nursing care is concerned, then, not only with the interrelationships of all the aspects of

128

the therapeutic plan but also with the interlocking effort of those who help administer the plan. As a result, she becomes aware of patterns of response within the individual as well as antecedent and consequent relationships within the organization or agency, and priorities or sequences. This awareness leads to a continuous investigation of the factors involved and decisions as to when, where, and by whom action is to be initiated.

Interrelationships and Patient Care

In the direct ministration of patient care, the nurse studies those factors which precipitate a crisis for the patient, how he modifies his behavior to handle a crisis, what are his prevailing patterns of response to a treatment or a drug, to his physical and social environment, to those in a helping role. How does he use his experiences? What kind of associations does he make which help him to predict his progress towards health? What resources does he recognize, and how does he use them?

Because the nurse is thoroughly acquainted with the total therapeutic plan, she has an opportunity to see the interrelationships of the parts of that plan. She can relate drug therapy to diet therapy, speech therapy to occupational therapy, physical therapy to rest therapy. She can appraise what is required of the patient in terms of physical effort, discomfort tolerance, and learning and concentration. She must make decisions with respect to timing, emphasis, and sequence. She decides when the patient needs assistance, support, encouragement, or sufficient frustration to help him mobilize his own powers.

Perhaps it is in the home setting that the nurse's coordinating functioning becomes most clear. Here the patient is in his natural habitat and the resources of the home and family are most apparent. Other resources are more remote, however, and she must rely heavily upon reporting, recording, conferring, and referring in order to make her decisions as to priorities, timing, and sequence. Not always is she herself ministering nursing care, but rather she helps family members to provide direct nursing care. Her skill in effecting a synchronization of human effort and in utilizing facilities which may be present in or added to the home environment may be called coordination.

When the patient is ambulatory and attending a clinic or receiving medical care in the physician's office, the nurse helps to interrelate the many single units of his care—drugs, diets, treatments, diagnostic measures, exercise, rest, and so on. Often she helps him examine what he knows and how he can use this knowledge. She helps him to work out schedules, self-checklists, to rearrange a physical setting, to reorganize the storage of personal belongings, to make easily accessible important telphone numbers, and so on. She helps the patient and family create a workable, functional situation, the product of coordination.

INTERRELATIONSHIPS WITHIN THE AGENCY PROVIDING PATIENT CARE

For some readers, an examination of the structure of the setting in which he or she works may help to clarify the concept of articulation which is the key to coordination. In today's hospital the increasing use of the nursing team and the emerging role of the clinical specialist, with its effect upon the role of the head nurse, the supervisor, and the nursing service administrator, have required the staff nurse to become more aware of relationships. These relationships, hopefully, are not concerned wholly with the traditional chain of command but with the matching of skills, expertise, and the requirements of the nursing situation. These requirements stem not only from the therapeutic plan for the patient's care, but from the human situation in which there is a wide range in kinds of response, interaction, and communication. Written descriptions of job responsibilities or organizational charts which diagram line and staff relationships often fail to reveal the relationships which have developed as people work together within the framework of an agency or institution. What has been called the formal and informal structure of an agency is a very real thing and can never be ignored.

Changes within the community agency providing public health nursing services have also forced the staff nurse to consider inter-relationships. With the inclusion of the licensed practical nurse, the homemaker, the home health aide, the public health aide, and the school nurse aide, the public health nurse is required to look at the articulation of effort and its effect upon family health.

Not only in the nursing community have new subdivisions or categories emerged, but within each of the other health professions as well. Consider the number of subcommunities within the hospital community. Each has its own particular characteristics which determine pattern of response and its interaction with other subcommunities.[2] Within the medical community, the interlocking of the efforts of intern, resident, chief of staff, and private physician, as well as those of the general practitioner, the internist, the surgeon, and other specialists, has great significance for the nurse; the synchronization of their planning vitally affects the patient's progress. Likewise, the community of social workers has its subgroups of medical, psychiatric, and group-work social workers each of which has a given setting with a structural uniqueness. Each agency—the hospital, the private clinic, and the family casework or welfare agency—has a framework which in turn affects the way in which the social worker relates to or articulates his efforts with those of other health worker communities, namely those of the physician and the nurse.

COMMUNICATION AS A MEANS
OF ESTABLISHING RELATIONSHIPS

Forces such as size of an organization or agency, sheer physical distance between individuals, the ignorance of common interests, as well as the emotional tensions which accompany any human endeavor far outweigh the forces which make articulation of effort possible.[3] Face-to-face communication is a major means of establishing relations between those who are to be involved in the receiving and giving of patient care. This communication needs to take place in the early phases of either an illness or employment experience. In the former, the early inclusion of the patient, the family, and other members of the nursing group at the time when information is being assembled helps immeasurably to establish a feeling of trust and confidence in each other. Directly or indirectly each will be involved in the use of that assembled information, and an early reciprocal relating of the factors in a situation sets the stage for the emergence of roles and responsibilities.

If the family knows to what use the information they give may be put, they begin to see their part as providers of that information and to become responsible for its completeness and accuracy. If the nurse's aide takes part in the early phase of assessment before the nursing diagnosis is made, then she perceives her contributions as significant and can be relied upon to observe and report the patient's symptoms. If the nurse is included in the planning of medical care and the evaluation of its outcomes, she becomes keenly aware that she holds a key position in describing the total patient situation. She becomes responsible for not only noting expected behavior but for observing the unusual and unanticipated occurrences. She shares information concerning the local effect of a treatment and the amount and kind of returns elicited; she also reports the total effect upon physical comfort, the relief of restlessness, the sense of pressure, and ease of movement. These examples of face-to-face communication in the early phases of assessment and planning and in the evaluation of immediate action contribute a great deal to the relationship of the parts to achieve an optimum quality of patient care.

When the nurse accepts a position within an agency providing health services, she needs information about the relationships already established within the agency. Today, some kind of orientation is usually provided. Too often, this orientation consists of telling her the line of command within the section of the organization in which she will function. In other words, she may be told to whom she is directly accountable and who is responsible to her. This information makes it possible for her to function immediately. However, she needs an early orientation not only to line but to staff relationships. For example, is there a staff council, and with what is it concerned? Are there nursing care conferences, and who is involved—the nursing team, the entire staff of the unit? Do the head nurse, the clinical specialist, the supervisor, the social worker, and the public health nurse coordinator ever participate, and in what way do they participate? What provisions are there for the planned conferences with the physician, the social worker, the physical therapist, or nutritionist? In the public health agency, what opportunity does the nurse have for conferring with the epidemiologist, the health educator, the public health engineer, or the public health officer or his deputy? Who is included in clinical rounds or in the evaluation of family situations and clinic services? Do members of the various health disciplines explore together new methods of treatment, review and expand their knowledge of disease entities, or examine some of the concepts pertinent to the underlying philosophy of patient care (rehabilitation, continuity and extension of care, teaching of patients, palliative care, etc.)?

Much has been written about the early exposure of the new nurse employee to the agency's philosophy of nursing care. Certainly this early exposure is essential, and a written statement of that philosophy should be available to her. How an understanding, then an appreciation, and finally a commitment to that philosophy develops, is often debated. To find a philosophy in action is far more meaningful than to see it in print. If the nurse sees in operation an organized plan for relating to others through the sharing of common interests and goals, face-to-face communication, and direct involvement in learning together and in decision-making, then the underlying philosophy of patient care becomes apparent to her. The written statement of that philosophy now has meaning to her. She has acquired a sense of partnership through verbal communication and persuasion in which relevant fact and informed opinion have been shared vertically and horizontally and the delegation of responsibility has been clearly defined.

REPORTING

Within her own sphere, the nurse performs some specific acts of communication: reporting, recording, conferring, and referring. The act of referring has been discussed at length in Chapter 8. Reporting, a form of oral communication, has long been emphasized as essential to the coordination of nursing care. However, its importance is magnified today when kinds of nursing personnel have increased so enormously. Paradoxically, the quality of the reporting has deteriorated, and often the amount of reporting has diminished. The written record which does not require face-to-face communication has often replaced most inadequately the oral report. Reporting requires the selection of pertinent and accurate information and the individuals with whom to share it. Pertinence is determined by the purpose of reporting and by the potential ability of the receiver of the information. If the purpose of reporting is to ensure a consistent approach to the problem of skin breakdown, then the details of the nursing measures taken to improve circulation, to relieve pressure, and to maintain a clean, dry environment should be shared with nursing personnel who have the skills to continue these measures. If the purpose of reporting is to arrive at a more concise appraisal of the patient's readiness for discharge, then information concerning the care the patient will need when he returns home would be shared with the family who have the ability to evaluate the home situation and to evaluate their own readiness to assume new responsibilities.

A designated time and place for reporting enhance the importance of reporting. In most agency settings, reporting occurs when there is a change in nursing personnel, when an interval of time has elapsed or whenever a significant episode in patient care has occurred. For example, in the hospital, traditionally, reporting from one nurse to another has occurred when a given period of assignment has elapsed, that is, when an eight-hour period of the day or night has transpired. In the public health agency, reporting is done at the end of a day of home visits or a period in a Well Child Conference or in a school. This reporting may be at the staff level or it may occur vertically in the hierarchy of command. Ideally, the time allotted for this reporting should be generous and should be regarded as time spent in giving nursing care. Too often, reporting time is replaced by "doing" time, because the latter is perceived as giving direct nursing care.

Frequently reporting takes place in hallways, across crowded desks, in linen closets and utility rooms, or sometimes in the patient's room. A provision in the architectural plan for a space set aside for face-to-face and written communication reinforces the important part reporting and recording plays in patient care. Architectural design expresses eloquently the philosophy and values of the designer or of those who have instructed him. This is demonstrated by the old dispensary with its large corridors for benches (the waiting area), its small cramped examining rooms, its open space where personal and vital information is taken. The same proof can be found in the older hospital or public health nursing agency where little or no room can be found for reporting, for group conferences, or where desks are jointly shared by several nurses. The provision of a place and the designation of a time for reporting does not guarantee that pertinent, accurate information will be given objectively to those who can best use it, but a setting places an emphasis upon the interchange of information and ideas.

RECORDING

Recording makes possible the preservation of information which may be exchanged in face-to-face communication. It also makes that information available to a greater number of people, and, if easily accessible to them, it results in more continuity of care. Because of the permanency of the record, judgment must be used as to what information should be preserved. This involves the consideration of how and by whom the information will be used. Unfortunately, writing skills which require selection and organization of content, have not been an integral part of the curricula in schools of nursing. Many nurses reject recording and do not perceive it as a part of nursing care. The growing insistence upon the record as a communication tool without the conscious development of recording skill has often resulted in the collection of insignificant material and the frustration of the nurse who does not see writing as part of doing. She often writes because something must appear on the record as legal evidence that she administered a medication or a treatment or that she did see the patient within a given interval of time. Forms have been developed for the purpose of this kind of checking. The nurse's record, then, may be delegated solely to the writing of observations of the patient's behavior, his responses to treatment and care, information given, and mutual planning between nurse and patient. In some agency settings, the tape recorder and the dictaphone have been introduced to relieve the nurse of the onus of writing. However, the exercise of judgment in selecting what information is pertinent for whom and the validation of that information can never become the responsibility of a mechanical device. Nor can the outcomes of communication, namely priority setting, decision-making, and evaluation, be relegated solely to any product of automation. In short, the cognitive skills of differentiation and interpretation of data, of summarization, prediction, and evaluation, begin to stand out sharply as undeniable skills which the nurse must possess if she is to administer comprehensive nursing care.

CONFERRING

Conferring is a form of communication which probably leads most directly to coordination. The outcome of a conference is a decision or decisions requiring action. If those decisions involve not only the persons who carry out the action but those whom the actions will affect, then the articulation of parts and the synchronization of forces is accomplished and coordination results.

What are the indications of a true conference? Data are pooled and shared. The significance of those data is determined by the interpretation given by each member of the conferring group. As interpretations are shared, they are aligned with the mutual goals of the group. Obstacles or problems may be identified. Gaps in information may become evident. Possible alternative action is considered; each action is examined in terms of its possible consequences and the facilities, time, and human resources needed to take that action. Eventually an action is selected, and responsibility with authority is delegated to some individual or individuals in the conferring group. When, where, and how the selected action is to be taken may be decided by the conferring group and may be part of the responsibility delegated to the action-taking individuals. Some decision is made as to how the outcome of the selected action will be judged. It is necessary to decide what evidence will be needed to determine whether the action selected is effective.

Throughout the entire act of conferring, deliberative, reflective thinking takes place. There is discussion, but a true conference is more than a discussion. The derivation of the term "discuss" is found in the Latin word, *discutere*: to scatter, to shake apart. Conferring puts together what has been examined and is synonymous with joint decision-making. The distinction between discussion and conference is often unclear. Many a so-called conference is simply a discussion, since no decision is made for further action.

The most outstanding characteristic of team or group nursing is said to be the daily team conference. If the reader can recall a nursing team conference she may have experienced, she should be able to identify the elements of a conference which were described in preceding paragraphs. For example, that the information shared by members of the team concerning the behavior of Mrs. Mills in interpreted by them to indicate Mrs. Mills' readiness to assume some responsibility in caring for her colostomy. A decision is made that tomorrow, the team leader, as she gives the daily colostomy irrigation, will discuss with Mrs. Mills her readiness. Similarly, the possibility of Mr. Sampson's ability to follow a special diet when he returns home is discussed in the nursing team conference. It is decided that Mr. Sampson's wife be invited to the next team conference to review with her the family diet, the feasibility of such a diet in terms of marketing facilities, food storage, and habitual cooking methods used in the home. In both examples, decisions reached were concerned with getting further information, with early involvement of those who will carry out the actions and those whom the actions will directly affect.

A conference may occur between the physician, the nurse, the social worker and the public health nurse, who reach the decision to request the visiting teacher to make weekly visit to an ill child. Such a decision is reached after considering the home situation and its potentials for continued bedrest with some opportunity for the child to cope with his anxiety over missed school work. Such a decision is tested out with the child to assure his willingness to participate in the plan.

It may be the psychiatric social worker in a community mental health center, the worker in a group-work agency, the public health nurse, and a patient recently discharged from a state hospital, who, through conferring together, decide that the former patient extend his group activities and spend fewer hours in the center. The group worker emerges as the member of the group who works most directly with him and keeps other members informed of his progress towards social rehabilitation.

In the school setting, a conference between the homeroom teacher, the school nurse, the parents, and the clinical psychologist may result ultimately in an effective coordination or relating of home and school resources. An informed cooperative group is then able to create an environment in which a child with a physical disability can develop socially, physically, and intellectually.

A final example may be cited in the work setting of an industry where the nurse, the foreman, and the safety engineer confer with respect to what measures can be taken to motivate workers to carry out safety regulations. What the workers may or may not know about the acids with which they work is considered thoughtfully, and a decision may be reached to set up a series of demonstrations by the foreman. Or it may be decided that protective devices are inadequate and the safety engineer is to explore what substitutes may be made.

Whoever participates in the conference or wherever it is held, the application of three principles will help ensure coordination as an ultimate outcome. First, some decision must be reached as to the next step or action to be taken. Second, the decision-making must involve those who will take the action decided upon and, if feasible, those whom the action will affect. Third, responsibility for and the authority to carry out the action must be delegated to an individual or individuals with some provision for evaluating the outcomes.

Whoever sees the need for conferring should initiate the process. That person may be the nurse's aide, the social worker, the nurse, or the teacher. However, since the primary concern in this volume is the administration of comprehensive nursing care, the emphasis here is upon the coordinating function of the nurse and her role as an initiator. Unfortunately, she often perceives herself as a participant in, but not the initiator of, a conference. She often sees herself as carrying out a decision, but not helping make that decision. With an increasing comprehension of the nature of nursing, she becomes more secure and gradually assumes a co-worker or colleague relationship. Frequently the shift from working *under* another's direction to working *with* that other comes about through her creating a situation in which this type of relationship is unavoidable.

Skill in Making Judgments

Decision-making requires the exercise of judgment. How does one develop judgment? What kind of experiences foster the growth of judgment? When is a judgment deemed good or wise? The exercise of judgment is one of the highest levels of cognitive skills. It requires the examination of what is known, a search for what is not known, the recognition and discrimination of shades and degrees of similarities and differences, the adding up of evidence, and finally a choice between alternatives which is based upon underlying values. Any experience in which the individual is asked to list the known facts and to identify the possible factors which may have produced a situation stimulates the deliberation which cultivates skill in judgment. Perhaps one of the outstanding characteristics of the professional practitioner is his or her ability to delay judgment until more evidence is obtained. Again, experiences which stimulate the individual to compare and contrast two or more situations or conditions help him to discriminate. Opportunities to weigh known facts or evidences and to choose an action and describe clearly what guided that choice develop a self-awareness which is essential to the development of judgment skill. When the action is taken and the consequences reviewed, the process of judgment making is completed, and the individual can then conclude whether the judgment was wise. Too frequently the individual is denied the privilege of taking the consequences of his judgment, and the improvement of future judgments is arrested.

In the performance of the coordinating function, the nurse is in a position to develop not only her own judgment skill but that of her co-workers. Specific experiences in the work setting afford opportunities to grow in this skill area. For example, teaching "rounds" stimulate the comparison and contrast of patient conditions, of response to nursing and medical treatments. The comparison and contrast of neighborhoods, home environments, and family groups helps the public health nurse discriminate between factors which predispose, precipitate, or perpetuate illness and disease or contribute to healthy adjustment and adaptation.

A series of so-called "bedside clinics" in which patients with identical disease diagnoses and similar or dissimilar nursing care problems or life-situations affords another excellent opportunity to practice discrimination. Family and patient studies which lead to some conclusions based on the assembled findings encourage the weighing of evidence required to reach a judgment. Too often the bedside clinic, the study of a patient or family, or the teaching rounds are remembered as student experiences but unheard of as a part of the experiences of the nurse-practitioner. She is described as much too busy; one wonders with what is she so busy?

The opportunity to choose the action to be taken and to abide by the consequences of that action is only possible when those facets of patient and family care in which the nurse makes the ultimate decision are clearly described. The traditional dependence of nursing action upon physician's orders has impeded the development of her judgment and decision-making skills.

Setting Priorities

One of the outcomes of the weighing of facts which is part of the judgment and decision-making processes is the setting of priorities. An order is given to whatever is being considered—patient or family needs, objectives or goals, actions to be taken. A sequence or succession is arranged which requires antecedent-consequent relationships. The selection of a beginning point is of tremendous importance in effecting the coordination of human and material resources. Motivation of human behavior is so complex, it is very difficult to establish precisely cause and effect relationships, but it is possible to determine what must take precedence. In previous chapters there has been discussion of the assessment of nursing needs, the setting of immediate and long-term nursing care objectives, and the planned sequence of nursing measures to be taken. In the coordination of the many facets of patient care, the nurse helps set priorities with respect to when and how much effort should be expended by which member or members of the inter- and intraprofessional group. In the latter, the nurse-administrator, whether she be team leader, district supervisor, or nursing service administrator, has to weigh the needs, the readiness, and skills of her staff with the needs, motivation, and the coping ability of the patient or family. The extent of her comprehension of the total human situation affects directly the setting of priorities.

Control Through the Delegation of Authority and Responsibility

Coordination is not complete without the supervision of the functioning of the whole organism. Just as the master gland in the human body receives messages and responds appropriately by inhibiting, stimulating, or maintaining the secretions of other glands, so the coordinating person exercises command and control over the operating units of the system. The operator of the master switchboard not only receives incoming messages and relays them, but he interprets those messages and transforms them into commands or directions to other recipients. Thus, by means of central control, reciprocal relationships are effected.

In any human situation, responsibility is concerned not only with accountability for something but to someone. Because of increasing emphasis upon freeing the individual to exercise initiative, to be creative, the delegation of responsibility must always signify the bestowing of the authority or prerogative to exercise judgment in the individual situation. Frequently authority is perceived as residing in a position or title: for example, the team leader, the supervisor, the physician, or the head nurse. If one considers responsibility as the counterpart of authority, it is evident that responsibility is given to the individual or individuals who possess the knowledge and the skill to apply it in a particular situation. In other words, authority resides in and grows out of the situation itself and the specific expertise it demands. The coordinating person who exerts central control needs to examine again and again the total community involved in the act of administration and to determine where true authority and responsibility lie.

A paradox seems to exist between the giving of responsibility and authority and the assumption of central control. Is not the latter equivalent to taking away what has been given? Is not the result personal frustration? The controversy is often phrased as decentralization versus centralization. In truth, there must be both. Without the latter, decentralization often deteriorates into fragmentation. Without the delegation of authority to the operational unit in a large system, the stultifying of individual initiative and the thwarting of potential leadership occur. In short, both central command and the delegation of accountability and authority to individuals at the operation level are necessary to accomplish coordination.

Supervision

Supervision is concerned with seeing the whole as well as the parts.

It is truly the overview which provides the individual at the operational level the perspective needed to see himself and the fruits of his labor as part of a unified whole. Supervision includes inspection of the process and product. However, it also makes available to the individual the background or context within which he operates. It requires not only guidance and direction, but also counseling and the giving of information. This may be sheer facts, concepts, or principles; the individual increases the resources needed to exercise the authority his work situation requires. With quality supervision, the individual can relate to and communicate with others and can integrate his thoughts, efforts, and accomplishments into a larger framework. This kind of supervision makes possible true self-realization and contributes largely to the internalization of control or discipline; this is a built-in order which is the sign of any functioning unit, whether it be the healthy human organism, the nurse-practitioner, or the nursing team administering comprehensive nursing care.

The function of supervision and the coordination which it implies may be difficult for the nurse who is action-oriented. She finds it much easier to give direct nursing care or to carry out an action rather than to see that another does so. Far greater control is needed for supervision. Greater sophistication and wisdom in the exercise of judgment leads to restraint. Eventually she is able to make it possible for another to give the quality of nursing care which she could provide and to excel her in the administration of comprehensive nursing care. She has learned that supervision is more than giving commands and directions and certainly more than inspecting.

Summary

The highly complex act of coordination relates the parts of a whole to each other in such a way that an order evolves out of their interdependece; this order synchronizes the efforts of each individual unit in such a way that a predetermined purpose is accomplished. A flow of communication within some kind of structure or organization is essential to the articulation of individual efforts. The balance and counterbalance of forces, both antagonistic and synergestic, is implied in such a structure. Skill in the exercise of judgment is essential in deciding the action to be taken, in setting priorities, in delegating responsibility and authority, in supervising, and in evaluating.

A few methods which the nurse uses in effecting coordination are reporting, recording, conferring, and referring. Orientation to the agency's philosophy of patient care and to the organization of the work situation, as well as to already established ways of relating and communicating is essential. Above all, effective coordination requires the active involvement of those who must carry out an action and who will be affected by the action.

Examples have been drawn from several settings—the hospital, community nursing agency, school, and industry—in which coordination of the efforts and resources of the patient, the family, nursing and other professional personnel, and the community group is imperative. Perhaps one of the greatest hopes of today's complex society is the increasing recognition that order and harmony may be brought about through coordination.

References

1. Follett, M.P. Dynamic Administration: The Collected Papers of Mary Parker Follett. Metcalf, H.C., and Norwick, L., eds. New York, Harper Brothers, 1942.
2. Burling, T., Lentz, E.M. and Wilson, R.N. Give and Take of the Hospital. New York, G.P. Putnam's Sons, 1956.
3. Tead, O. The Art of Administration. New York, McGraw-Hill Book Company, 1951.

11

Evaluating Nursing Care

Evaluation is concerned with determining the worth or value of a product and the process by which it is produced. An outcome and the act of achieving that outcome are examined.

The estimation of the worth of a product implies the initial acceptance of some kind of standards. It is upon these standards that the evaluation of the product's quality is based. Was the intent of the act to produce a desirable change in human behavior—for example, in understanding, in attitude, or in performing certain skills? Without the conscious consideration of the original intent of the producer, the evaluator has no direction and evaluation becomes capricious and purposeless. What was necessary to produce the product, to achieve the desired outcome? What kind of materials were needed; what techniques had to be used; what kind of safeguards had to be observed; what supervision was provided; what decisions were required?

If evaluation of both the product and the process occurs, goals or objectives may be reaffirmed, modified, or rearranged, or new goals may be set up. Again, the process may be facilitated by refocusing the emphasis on some aspect of the coordinated effort of the workers. Perhaps the safeguards were judged to be sufficient, but the motivation of the worker to use such safeguards needed improvement. The kind of supervision provided must be more guided. The readiness of the worker to assume certain responsibilities and authority must be assessed more carefully.

Evaluation begins when goals are determined. At that moment, the obtainable evidence or data that a desired outcome has been attained must be described. From the moment that a direction is taken, evaluation is continuous. It occurs at the site of action, during the operation, with the final outcome in mind.

Obviously, to evaluate the product and the process, three requisites must be met: there must be 1) a knowledge of the initial intent or objectives; 2) a knowledge of the basic materials, resources, and facilities available; and 3) evidence of the progress made in using the resources to attain the predetermined goal. Two points of reference are needed in order to estimate progress, the goal to be reached and the starting point or baseline.

THE PRODUCT AND THE PROCESS

The central goal of comprehensive nursing care is to restore or to promote a state of being in which the individual or family serves his or their best and lives as fully as possible. Prevention of disease is a part of that goal, but the fostering or nurturing of well-being goes beyond prevention of disease. In other words, the product to be evaluated is some desirable change in the patient's or family's behavior—improved kidney function, a stabilized blood pressure, an acceptance of physical limitations, a skill in using a new means of locomotion, a skill in performing the activities of daily living, increased food intake, insight as to how the illness experience can be used constructively, restored ability to relate effectively to one's social environment.

The process by which the ultimate goal of comprehensive nursing care is reached involves the effective relating of the giver to the recipient of that care, what Ida Orlando[1] calls the deliberative approach of one human being to another in which exploration and the testing of interpretations occur. This leads to assessing what is needed and what can be provided, setting up immediate goals which the giver and recipient share and accept, and deciding what action can be taken and what resources can be used. The implementation of that decision becomes part of the nursing process, along with the evaluation of the consequences, the decisions reached, the goals set up, and the assessment initially made. Engaged in the process is the individual giving nursing care who may belong to any of the many categories of nursing personnel. The comprehensiveness of the care depends upon the comprehension of those who give it directly or who provide for the care given; the nature of the nursing process reflects the comprehension of those who provide nursing care.

An attempt has been made in previous chapters to describe the dynamics of the nursing process. Any attempt to evaluate nursing care will not only include an estimate of the desirable change in the behavior of the recipient, but also the behavioral changes in the giver. Growth in the giver's comprehension of what nursing care is (a change in cognitive and affective behavior) and in his psychomotor skills becomes an accepted and acceptable goal.

THE BASELINE

In evaluating the outcome or product of nursing care, those desired changes in patient and family behavior, where does one find the baseline necessary to estimate the progress made? The nursing history taken on admission, the so-called "intake" interview (conducted in early home visits), and the recording of initial observations of behavior serve to establish a baseline which describes that patient or family at the time the process of effecting changes in his or their behavior began. What did he know of his disease condition when nursing care was first instituted? What, if any, motion was displayed in a paralyzed limb when the nurse made her first visit to the home? What did the mother disclose as to her feelings about this pregnancy when she began her visits to the prenatal clinic? What does the patient report as his daily diet, his food preferences during those first days of contact with the nurse? What was the patient's response to other patients when he first entered the psychiatric unit?

Unless the nurse has a clear picture of the patient's physiologic, psychosocial behavior at the onset of nursing care, no estimate can be made of the extent to which his behavior has changed. Mr. Evans, at the time of admission, had no flexion in the fingers of his right hand. Five days later he could grasp and partially squeeze a face-cloth but could not unscrew the cap on his shaving cream tube. He has made far more progress towards his goal than has Mr. Bowman who, on admission, could squeeze a face-cloth dry but cannot yet unscrew the cap of his shaving cream tube.

The baseline necessary to evaluate the characteristics of the nursing process is found in the initial appraisal of the comprehension of those who give nursing care. This appraisal includes some insight as to what that individual believes nursing to be. What has been her preparation, experience, and former performance? Has the individual had some kind of orderly preparation in which her needs as a learner have been considered? Has her preparation been tailored to the needs of the immediate situation in which she is to perform some specific task? Has her experience been limited in scope and in depth or restricted to a specific setting, to the nursing care of patients with a certain combination of nursing needs?

This inventory provides some kind of prediction as to what extent and in what way the individual can engage in the nursing process. The baseline is actually established when, in the initial assignments, the individual has the opportunity to demonstrate his ability to assess nursing needs, to select and carry out actions to meet nursing needs in terms of priority, and to continue or modify actions in relation to the effect upon the patient and family. Has the new nurse's preparation been primarily in the service or work situation in which she has been assigned a job to be done? Has she been instructed as to the procedures which are to be carried out with a minimum of background knowledge as to the purposes of the procedures and the expected outcomes? Or has she had an extended preparation both in and away from the clinical setting in which she has had an opportunity to study human behavior, to relate action to purpose and outcome? During such preparation, she may have cared for a few selected patients but never had the opportunity to provide for the care of a group of patients, to give leadership to co-workers in a nursing situation. Does she evidence a knowledge of the disease condition, the patient's life situation, or a responsiveness to the patient's behavior? To what extent does she show an ability to coordinate the resources available to her and the patient and family? With this initial inventory of the nurse's preparation, experience, and competencies, the evaluator establishes a baseline which will help her estimate the extent to which the nursing process has been used.

GATHERING THE EVIDENCE

If desirable change in the behavior of either the recipient or the giver or both is to be estimated, then evidence is found in individual behavior. Human behavior, the mode of response to internal and external stimuli, is made up of thinking, feeling, and doing. It is both physiologic and psychosocial in nature. Behavior is both covert and overt. Overt behavior is observable and provides objective evidence for evaluation. What can be seen, heard, felt, tasted, and smelled gives the data which, when assembled in organized form, lead to conclusions as to whether the goal was reached. The evidence must be sufficient in amount and relevant to the objective or goal. It must be accurate and submitted to classification by several judges in order to be reliable.

If the immediate objective of nursing care is to relieve the patient's constipation, what evidence will be sought to determine whether that objective was attained? The nurse will consider amount, consistency, color of the stool, and the ease and regularity (in accordance with the individual's regular pattern) of the act of evacuation. This series of indicators can be used in estimating the relief of constipation. With sufficient evidence submitted, if possible, to several judges, a conclusive judgment can be reached.

How does one know that healing has been promoted? Several indicators come to mind: the increase in granulation tissue, the color and turgor of the skin surrounding the wound, the decrease in sero-sanguinious discharge, the patient's expression of an itching or "pulling" sensation. Repeated clinical observation has yielded a sufficient number of instances or facts to provide indicators of physiologic behavior which are called physical signs and symptoms. The reader easily recalls the indicators that could be used to determine whether shock has been prevented, blood pressure has been stabilized, fluid electrolyte balance has been restored, the nutritional state improved. In estimating the progress made in attaining the desirable behavior, observable evidence can be obtained. The functioning of the systems of the body, what Bowen[2] refers to as cellular communities and subcommunities, produces overt evidence which, with increasing refinement of data-collecting instruments, is now available in making an evaluation, a prognosis, a prescription. A list of such overt evidence would include not only waste or excretory products, secretions, respiratory and circulatory rates, but also electrical impulses, energy output, and so on.

Many of the objectives of nursing care are concerned with changes in psychosocial behavior. For example, an objective may be to relieve preoperative anxiety; to relieve pain; to help the patient cope with a change in his body-image; to help the family accept the limitations of an invalid, partially senile father; to motivate an adult worker to use the occupational health services available to him; or to help a young mother understand the developmental tasks of her four-year-old son. The overt or observable evidences of change in the degree of anxiety, in the amount and kind of pain, in self-image, in acceptance, motivation, and understanding, are less well-described or even identified. On the other hand, the nurse may be less aware of and therefore less responsive to the indicators of pain, anxiety, readiness to learn, and tendencies to act in certain ways. Is she aware of the many ways in which anxiety, grief, pain, motivation, rejection, and acceptance are expressed? Has she as a clinician accumulated a series of instances of individual behavior from which she can develop a useful list of indicators to be used in evaluating change in behavior? Only through repeated, carefully directed or disciplined observation of the behavior of patients in the hours immediately preceding surgery, of patients who are experiencing pain, of the mother's handling of her first newborn, of families caring for some member with a long-term illness, does she extend the range of evidence which can be used to evaluate the amount and kind of change in behavior. She is then able to use the indicators to determine low, moderate, or high anxiety and to judge whether the pain is now absent, more tolerable, or less tolerable to the patient.

Indicators of change in the characteristics of the nursing process also need to be identified if the behavioral change of the giver of nursing care is to be evaluated. A faculty group attempted to identify what behavior indicates average, above average, and considerably above average assessment of patient and family needs, definition of immediate and long-term goals, use of resources, and so on. Table 1 relates the result of their efforts. The behavior of the senior student was then observed throughout the period of her clinical experience for specific instances which fell within one of the three lists of indicators. A judgment could then be made as to the amount of progress the student had demonstrated in the several phases of the nursing process. The reader is reminded that the faculty were informed of the kind of behavior the student had demonstrated in the previous clinical setting, so that a baseline was present.

METHODS AND EVALUATIVE TOOLS

Observation

Observation, questioning and measurement have been used as aids to evaluation in nursing situations. Measurement has generally been confined to clinical measurement. Within the team of health workers, the nurse ranks high in her observation skill. Her early training emphasizes the observation of physiologic behavior. She must note the color of mucous membranes, the gait of the patient, the color of the urine, the position of a limb; she feels the pulse, the turgor of the skin, the contraction of a muscle; she smells the odor of the breath, perspiration, discharge from a wound; and she hears the fetal heartbeat, the patient's breathing. Through the intelligent use of all her senses, she gathers a wealth of data related to physiologic behavior.

Thoughts, feelings, and attitudes are expressed in observable nonverbal and verbal behavior. The evaluator looks for changes in posture, facial expression, gestures, as well as flushing, paling, moistening lips, the rubbing of moist palms. She notes what is said as well as what is not said, the rate and pressure of speech, the inflection and volume of the voice. She is well aware of opening and closing sentences, the unfinished sentence, the association of ideas, the sudden change of subject, and any prevailing theme in the conversation.

If process is being evaluated, then the behavior not only of the recipient of nursing care but of the giver of nursing care must be observed. The nurse is observed in the act of relating to the patient, to visitors, and to co-workers. The observer notes what is reported and recorded, what questions are asked of whom and at what time. She

TABLE 1. Guide for Evaluation of Student's Achievement in Public Health Nursing*

Main Objective: To apply and develop further nursing skills in helping selected families meet their health needs in the family and community setting through:

Sub-Objective 1—Increased ability in assessing health needs

(C)†	(B)†	(A)†
1. Selects key information from the record or referral, to appraise health needs of each member of family and of family as a whole.	⟶ ⟶	⟶ ⟶
2. Recognizes that her own experiences determine her attitude toward health and will therefore color her evaluation of the family situation.	⟶ ⟶	⟶ ⟶
3. Considers the socioeconomic, cultural, and educational factors in the family situation.	⟶ ⟶	⟶ ⟶
4. Gathers from the family information which is essential to determine the existing or potential health needs.	⟶ ⟶	⟶ ⟶
5. Indicates that she considers the various origins of health needs.	⟶ ⟶	⟶ ⟶

*Developed by faculty in the Department of Public Health Nursing in the College of Nursing, University of Bridgeport in 1968-69. Permission granted by faculty members: Nelliana Best, Ruth Canty, Betty Ford and Hannah Russell.

† C = average achievement, B = above average, A = considerably above average. Please note that some behavior statements appear on more than one level, as indicated by extended arrows. Other statements are modified at another level to indicate advanced cognitive, affective, or psychomotor skill.

6. Seeks from a variety of sources (literature, knowledgeable people) knowledge to increase her awareness of potential health needs. $\longrightarrow$ $\longrightarrow$
7. Assesses attitudes of family members toward health. $\longrightarrow$ $\longrightarrow$

8. Assesses the degree of the family's perception of its health needs.
9. Estimates the knowledge of family members of good health practices.

Sub-Objective 2—Increased ability in developing plans based on an analysis of family's needs and resources

(C)	(B)	(A)
1. Recognizes and uses her own resources (i.e., knowledge of good health practices, disease conditions, community resources, and ability to use her relationship with the family.		
2. Accepts responsibility for planning with family for periods between nursing visits.	$\longrightarrow$ $\longrightarrow$	$\longrightarrow$ $\longrightarrow$
3. Helps family understand its health needs.	3.1 Helps family accepts its health needs.	3.2 Helps family evaluate their progress toward the goals.
4. Helps family set up attainable goals (short- and long-term).		
5. Demonstrates sensitivity to potential	$\longrightarrow$ $\longrightarrow$	$\longrightarrow$ $\longrightarrow$

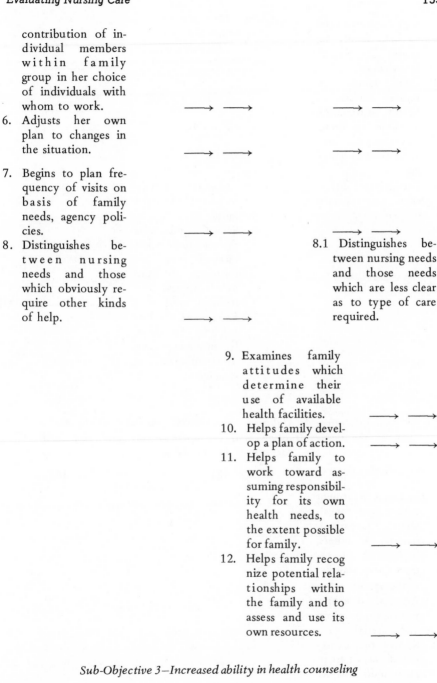

contribution of individual members within family group in her choice of individuals with whom to work.

6. Adjusts her own plan to changes in the situation.

7. Begins to plan frequency of visits on basis of family needs, agency policies.

8. Distinguishes between nursing needs and those which obviously require other kinds of help.

    8.1 Distinguishes between nursing needs and those needs which are less clear as to type of care required.

9. Examines family attitudes which determine their use of available health facilities.

10. Helps family develop a plan of action.

11. Helps family to work toward assuming responsibility for its own health needs, to the extent possible for family.

12. Helps family recognize potential relationships within the family and to assess and use its own resources.

Sub-Objective 3—Increased ability in health counseling

    (C)   (B)   (A)

1. Shows a good background of reliable health knowledge.

2. Seeks opportunities to help family increase its health knowledge.   ⟶ ⟶   ⟶ ⟶

3. Helps family appraise sources of health information available to them.   ⟶ ⟶   ⟶ ⟶

4. Capitalizes on family interest in learning.   ⟶ ⟶   ⟶ ⟶

5. Recognizes difference in capacity to learn.

5.1 Stimulates family to want to learn more.   ⟶ ⟶

6. Selects and uses the content and method most appropriate to family's readiness and learning needs.   ⟶ ⟶

7. Evaluates her teaching by closely observing family's progress in learning.   ⟶ ⟶

Sub-Objective 4—Ability to give skilled nursing care to the sick in the home situation, and to supervise care given by family or others in the home

(C)	(B)	(A)
1. Performs treatment with regard for a) safety of patient, family, and others, b) comfort of patient and family, c) therapeutic effectiveness, d) economy of time, effort, and materials.		
2. Knows the expected effects of treatment and medicines which the patient is receiving.	⟶ ⟶	⟶ ⟶
3. Anticipates possible complications or af-	⟶ ⟶	⟶ ⟶

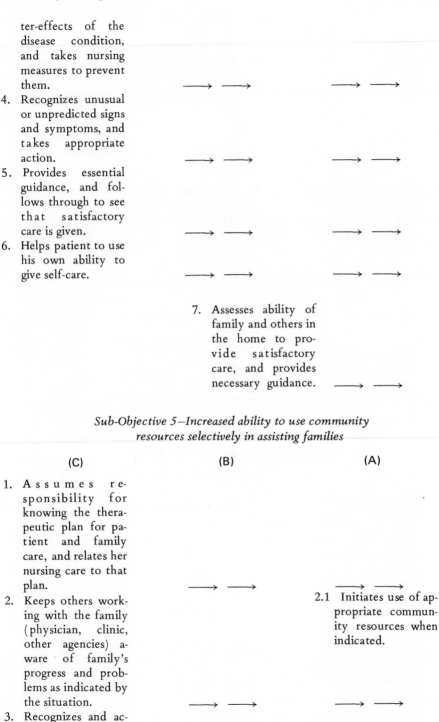

ter-effects of the disease condition, and takes nursing measures to prevent them.
4. Recognizes unusual or unpredicted signs and symptoms, and takes appropriate action.
5. Provides essential guidance, and follows through to see that satisfactory care is given.
6. Helps patient to use his own ability to give self-care.

7. Assesses ability of family and others in the home to provide satisfactory care, and provides necessary guidance.

Sub-Objective 5—Increased ability to use community resources selectively in assisting families

(C) (B) (A)

1. Assumes responsibility for knowing the therapeutic plan for patient and family care, and relates her nursing care to that plan.
2. Keeps others working with the family (physician, clinic, other agencies) aware of family's progress and problems as indicated by the situation.

2.1 Initiates use of appropriate community resources when indicated.

3. Recognizes and accepts the purpose, functions, and limitations of agency.

3.1 Interprets agency services meaningfully.

3.2 Knows the purpose, functions, limitations of most commonly needed health and welfare agencies in the community.

4. Uses commonly accepted procedure of referral in working with other agencies.

4.1 Helps family select those resources which best meet their needs.

4.2 Coordinates her work with that of other agencies to promote integrated and continuous care of the family.

5. Evaluates the effectiveness of family's use of a community resource.

⟶ ⟶   ⟶ ⟶

Sub-Objective 6—Some ability to use records effectively as a tool for both service and evaluation

(C)   (B)   (A)

1. Writes all records, including daily report, accurately, legibly, and with good grammatical form.

2. Clearly shows, in her service record, her observations, information gathered, her nursing action, immediate result, and plan for next visit.

⟶ ⟶   ⟶ ⟶

3. Records in family record her contacts with physician and other workers concerned with care of family.

⟶ ⟶   ⟶ ⟶

4. Keeps records up-to-date and available to those who need them.

    4.1 Records a complete nursing care plan, including long term as well as short term objectives. ⟶ ⟶

5. Uses the record as a major tool in revealing changes in situation, in providing continuity of care, and evaluating service. ⟶ ⟶

6. Clearly shows in service record what are the ideas, decisions, and actions of family. ⟶ ⟶

7. Writes summaries showing services rendered, progress made by family, and future plan.

    7.1 Writes summaries of service which show evaluation of situation encountered.

    7.2 Writes summaries of service which show thoughtful evaluation of situation encountered.

Sub-Objective 7—Increased ability to develop and to maintain a helpful relationship with families and co-workers

(C)	(B)	(A)
1. Creates an atmosphere in which both nurse and family are comfortable in discussing problems.		
2. Shows beginning understanding that people change slowly and will only accept the help they want.	⟶ ⟶	⟶ ⟶
3. Uses a non-judgmental approach.	3.1 Truly invests herself in people, giving warmth and support but recog-	⟶ ⟶

nizing the degree to
which she can be
helpfully involved.

4. Has the courage to
express an opinion,
yet is tolerant of
the point of view of
others.

⟶ ⟶

⟶ ⟶

5. Keeps agency per-
sonnel currently in-
formed of signifi-
cant aspects of fam-
ilies under her care.

6. Shows loyalty to
the agency, and
consideration of its
personnel, both in
the agency and in
community con-
tacts.

⟶ ⟶   ⟶ ⟶

⟶ ⟶   ⟶ ⟶

*Sub-Objective 8—Increased ability to evaluate realistically
one's own ability and performance, to use supervision constructively,
and to assume appropriate responsibilities for her personal conduct*

(C)   (B)   (A)

1. Sees supervision as
a learning experi-
ence.

1.1 Recognizes her
own assets and limi-
tations when mea-
suring progress to-
ward accepted
goals.

⟶ ⟶

2. Follows through on
suggestions by try-
ing out mutually ac-
cepted ideas.

3. Questions sugges-
tions if unable to
see their usefulness
in the particular sit-
uation.

⟶ ⟶   ⟶ ⟶

3.1 Identifies areas
where particular
help may be
needed. Seeks nec-
essary assistance
from appropriate
sources.

⟶ ⟶

4. Appears well
groomed.

5. Dresses appropriate-
ly for the weather
and the specific ac-

⟶ ⟶   ⟶ ⟶

tivities to be carried
out.
6. Uses time effective-
ly in the agency.
7. Carries out health
practices to main-
tain physical health
and emotional sta-
bility.

$\longrightarrow \longrightarrow$ $\longrightarrow \longrightarrow$

$\longrightarrow \longrightarrow$ $\longrightarrow \longrightarrow$

$\longrightarrow \longrightarrow$ $\longrightarrow \longrightarrow$

observes the nursing care objectives which are stated in the nursing care plan or presented in nursing care conferences. The amount and kind of participation in these conferences provides significant data. The observer sees what use is made of authoritative information which is available in the ward library, the pharmacopeia text, and so on. Likewise, techniques used in giving treatments and medications and in ministering to the physical needs of the patient are observed. The setting of priorities is demonstrated in many ways. One must note, for example, in what sequence does the individual order her activities. Does she give care first to the most acutely ill patient, to the patient who expresses verbally the most discomfort, or to the patient whose "routine" care can be given most quickly? Does she preface the home visit by reviewing the record? Does she schedule the home visit at the time when key members in the family group will be at home?

An observation guide helps to focus the observer's attention on what to look for. The evaluator needs to know what she is looking for, what indicates the desirable behavior which she is helping the recipient or the giver to attain. Sometimes checklists have been used as observation guides. Great care should be taken in preparing a checklist. A period of repeated unstructured observation needs to precede the final checklist. If not, the results of the checklist are restricted, since the number of indicators is much too limited.

David Fox,[3] who has worked closely with those engaged in research in nursing, points out some of the difficulties in the use of the observation method in collecting data for the purpose of evaluation. The presence of the observer alters the situation, and its naturalness becomes debatable. Even in the nurse-patient situation, the patient's behavior in response to the nurse may vary greatly from his behavior when alone. Frequently the nurse finds some opportunity to observe the patient when he is alone or in some interpersonal situation which does not include the nurse. However, if her contacts with the patient are frequent and sufficient in number, the probability that the patient's behavior become more typical is high. When both patient and nurse are being observed, the presence of the observer most certainly changes the situation. The parties observed attempt to find a reason for presence of the observer, and their awareness that they are under scrutiny changes what is being observed. The observer, in turn, cannot be sure what he is observing.[3]

One-way vision mirrors, the audio tape recorder, and more recently the closed-circuit television which makes possible video taping, have eliminated the presence of the observer. David Fox and others have emphasized the ethical issue of the individual's right to know that he is being observed.[3] There is widespread agreement that the individual give consent to the use of such devices. Interestingly enough, when consent has been given, the individual often recalls his discomfort during the period of observation. In one instance, a graduate student, having gained the consent of a family to use the tape recorder during home visits, shared the recording with the family, and together they analyzed the process and the outcome of the visit. The real source of discomfort—how the observations would be used—was removed, and the family became active participants in the act of evaluation.

The team leader who participates with team members in giving direct care to the patient has the advantage of being perceived as an integral part of the nursing situation. The reason for her presence is never a matter of conjecture. On the other hand, she may find her attention divided or that she has attempted too much. However, what is gained in demonstrating her commitment to the objectives of comprehensive nursing care may outweigh what is lost in terms of the extent of her observations.

Observation is highly selective. The sensory intake of the observer is determined by her background and experiences, by her phenomenologic field. Even though the same observation guide is used, no two observers will make identical observations, nor will any one observer see all that there is to be seen or hear all that is there to be heard. Therefore, in evaluating the product and the process—the behavioral change in the recipient and the giver of nursing care—more than one observer is essential. All should have similar backgrounds and experiences, and all should be well aware of what they are looking for. The number of similar observations made by several observers within a given period of time will help to establish the reliability of the judgment made.

QUESTIONING

Questioning is a method of collecting data which is particularly helpful in freeing the respondent to express himself and in obtaining information which may provide insight as to how he thinks and feels. However, questioning gives the evaluator only the verbal response, never the action. The verbal response may describe an action, either one completed in the past or to be taken in the future, but the act itself is never there.

When desirable change in covert rather than overt behavior is the objective, questioning is an excellent method for collecting evidence. Questions may be asked in a face-to-face situation in the course of a purposeful conversation. They may be written as in a questionnaire, or used indirectly in a checklist, a critical incident, or anecdotal record. The interviewing technique is by far the most difficult one used in the questioning method, but it probably yields the most conclusive evidence. The interviewer and the interviewee are influenced not only by the question asked and the response given, but by each other—age, sex, socioeconomic class, ethnic background, dress, facial expressions, and so on. The attitude of the interviewer, as well as the physical setting in which the interview takes place, affects the responses.

There are many kinds of questions, some of which need to be avoided if the evidence is to be as objective as possible and free of the bias or prejudice of the interview. Obviously, a question which implies the answer desired cannot be used to evaluate the behavior of the respondent: "The pain is less now, isn't it?" "What's the baby doing that's new?"

Questions which require yes or no answers are useful if factual information is needed and are best reserved for the written questionnaire or the checklist. An open-ended question which may provoke a wide range of responses is preferable when seeking insight as to feeling and thought processes; it lends itself to the unstructured interview. Often the open-ended question provokes a depth of response which can be explored in the interview. On the other hand, the yes or no question, or one which invites a fairly superficial opinion or judgment, can be used in the written questionnaire. At time of discharge, patients are sometimes asked to check on a questionnaire a statement which best expresses their opinion of some aspect of their hospital experience. The summary of patients' opinions has been found to be very different from that of responses given in interviews at the time of discharge when the patient was asked, "How did you feel about . . . ?" Some questions threaten the patient by seeming to invade his private world, to press him into revealing that which should be inaccessible to another human being, to corner him into giving reasons for his behavior. Some questions include a psychologically charged word or phrase. Depending upon the individual's experience and background, such words or phrases as "discharge," "training," or "insecure" may distort the response.

The interviewer must be highly sensitive to another individual's frame of reference. The question enters at some point in the field of the respondent's thinking. The response is determined not only by what was taken in, but by how it was perceived. Sometimes, it is wise for the interviewer to indicate his frame of reference to the respondent: "How are things going? I mean with respect to the new diet."

Skill in selecting shared words or phrases and in using appropriate figures of speech is important in formulating questions. Failure to use shared words frequently emphasizes those barriers between interviewer and interviewee which arise from differences in social and economic status, education, life experiences, and ethnic background. Nurses who work with families in certain neighborhoods, districts, or with children within a certain developmental period, or with workers in a given industry or occupational setting, become highly conversant with the many colloquialisms and jargon of these particular groups. They have a language in common with those with whom they work.

Two tools which require indirect questioning have been used as aids in evaluating change in the comprehension of the giver of nursing care. The critical incident and the anecdotal record have been requested of the nurse to reproduce an incident which she perceives as critical in its effect upon the patient or family, or to record an incident which she finds significant for herself in terms of success or failure in attaining desired goals.

An incident in which the patient or family was affected favorably or unfavorably is described. Then the nurse is asked to select from her own experience a similar incident, to describe what led up to the incident, who was involved, what happened, and what were the consequences. If a sufficient number of incidents are described, the evaluator can gain considerable insight as to what the respondent perceives as critical as well as to a wider view of what the experiences of the respondent have been. More data concerning the latter's evaluation or appraisal of nursing action and nurse-patient interaction can be acquired than by means of direct questioning.

The anecdote or brief account of the circumstances serves as a kind of "candid camera" shot which preserves a happening. Any evaluation of the happening is excluded and an effort is made to avoid the use of modifying words such as kindly, rapidly, gentle, embarrassed, and so on. A series of anecdotes written at frequent intervals over a prolonged period of time may provide a pattern of behavior, change in behavior, and insight as to the individual's personal frame of reference. If an anecdotal record is kept by both the evaluator and the staff member, then shared and compared, there may be a wide variance between what each perceives as important or significant in the nursing process. Early anecdotes give a baseline, succeeding anecdotes show change, and the final anecdotes serve to determine progress made. Difference in goals and in the priority placed upon mutual goals may be recognized and resolved.

The writing and sharing of anecdotes and critical incidents require time, and a period should be designated during which material is accumulated. When used to refine the nursing process, these techniques have fostered reflective, deliberate evaluation and have added greatly to the data which the questioning method may obtain.

MEASUREMENT

The nurse has fallen heir to the measurement techniques used in the various fields of medicine and in teaching. She uses the clinical thermometer and the sphygmomanometer; she measures the pulse, respiratory rate, fluid intake and output; she uses a variety of laboratory tests to estimate the adequacy of physiological functions. She has become more and more involved in diagnostic and evaluative techniques. The rapid development of diagnostic and intensive care units in the hospital has led to increased skill in the evaluation of the patient's physiologic behavior. With the increasing emphasis on evaluation in rehabilitation medicine, the nurse has participated in grading or rating the patient's psychomotor skills, his ability to carry out the activities of daily living, his locomotor abilities, and his response to sensory stimuli.

However, the measurement of covert behavior—affective as well as the upper levels of cognitive behavior—is still undeveloped.[4] Paper and pencil tests have been used to determine the patient's knowledge of specific facts or procedures. In the clinic situation, individuals have been tested on their knowledge of desirable health practices, of the anatomy and physiology of the body, and of procedures to carry out. The widespread use of quizzes in mass media has helped to make such testing seem appropriate and therefore acceptable to the patient. However, the evaluation of cognitive behavior at the level of under-standing (analysis, interpretation, synthesis, the use of evidence to make a judgment) is still very difficult, not only because of the lack of measurement tools and techniques, but because what is to be measured is still unclear. Essay questions, situational tests, and cause-effect questions have been used in teaching situations but often with lack of clarity as to what is being measured and considerable disagreement as to the worth of the evidence.

The measurement of affective behavior, whether at the levels of awareness, emotional readiness, attention-giving response, values or appreciations, and attitudes, is still in its infancy. Evaluation of affective behavior is generally confined to the evidence gathered by the gross observation of overt or psychomotor behavior and by questioning. Skilled clinicians have used both verbal and nonverbal projective techniques; for example, the uncompleted sentence, the inkblot, or the vague picture or cartoon are used to stimulate responses which may help the clinician make an inference or prediction with respect to behavior, but he is not concerned with the evaluation of behavior.

In some of the efforts in nursing research to evaluate changes in attitude and differences in cultural values, rating and rank order scales have been used, as well as the Q sort. Rarely have these techniques been used in ongoing practice situation. It may be advisable to consider their use in the work setting. The nurse's ability to set priorities may be evaluated by asking her to place in rank order a series of nursing actions which could be taken in a given nursing situation. Given a behavioral description of several hypothetical patients, she may be asked to justify her rating of each patient as most likely, likely, or least likely to change his behavior. Some estimate can then be made of the nurse's ability to assess and make a judgment. In other words, the use of the single or multiple choice question, the matching of items, the completion of sentences, and the ranking and rating of given items need not be confined to the formal classroom setting but in many instances could be used appropriately in the clinical situation to evaluate those upper levels of thinking and feeling which must be employed in the giving of comprehensive nursing care.

THE ANTECEDENT-CONSEQUENT RELATIONSHIP

In evaluating patient care, there has always been a query as to what brought about the desirable change in behavior. What was done, by whom, and when, that helped Mr. Edwards regain his speech? Was it the nurse's careful explanation of what could be done to relieve immediate postoperative discomfort that resulted in no postoperative nausea or vomiting and a minimum of pain-relieving medications? The constant search for what had to precede in order for the desired outcome to occur has focused attention upon the act of nursing intervention or those nursing measures which were selected to direct the patient's course towards a desired goal.

When the nurse meets with success repeatedly, she generalizes and adopts that nursing measure or act of intervention to be used in similar situations. She formulates a guide to action or a principle which can be used again and again. The principle is based upon empirical evidence, repeated observation and experience. However, unless she identifies other factors in the patient or family situation which can and may contribute to the desired outcome, she cannot safely predict that the "tried-and-true" nursing measure should be used universally. The complexity of individual behavior and the integrity of the interpersonal situation make it extremely difficult, if not impossible, to control rigidly those other factors which may have brought about recovery or improvement in the patient's condition, or those which may have prevented disease. In the terminology of research, an antecedent-consequent relationship is hard to establish. Was it the resolution of the blood clot in the brain, the patient's high level of motivation, or the nurse's continual reinforcement of the retraining instituted by the speech therapist? Was it the surgeon's or the anesthetist's visit the night before surgery, the patient's ability to cope with his anxiety because he had done his worrying before he entered the hospital, the nurse's deliberative, exploratory approach to the patient preoperatively when she made it possible for him to express his concerns,[5] or simply time spent by one nurse with the patient in that period before he received a sedative?

In recent years, studies have been made, replicated, and modified to identify more conclusively the independent variable in nursing care which determines the desired change in behavior. With continuing disciplined inquiry, it may be possible for the evaluation of nursing intervention to become more reliable. The guides to action which the nurse uses may become based upon the results of scientific investigation rather than upon practice or experience. Success becomes less a gamble and more a safe prediction.

SEARCH AND RESEARCH

The root of inquiry lies in concern. Expressed concern provides a clue as to where the individual may begin his exploration of factors in a situation or of aspects of behavior which have not been recognized. The nurse may be stimulated to return to the clinical situation to observe more closely and to search for indicators of categories of behavior—anxiety, anger, pain, fear, change in self-image, grief, guilt, disorientation. Unless she is aware of its many manifestations, how can she determine that anxiety has been reduced or change in body-image has been accepted? She may return to the clinical situation or to the family home to identify factors which precipitate or perpetuate undesirable behavior. As her observation becomes more controlled or directed, she is ready to select an appropriate action, to try it out again and again with deliberate, conscious attention to the outcome.

Systematic, disciplined inquiry is one of the traits of professional practice. Through her disciplined observation, her deliberate selection of nursing action, and her recognition of change in behavior, the nurse-practitioner can make a very real contribution to research, an endeavor which requires highly specialized skills. In turn, she can become an intelligent consumer of the product of research if she can evaluate critically the conclusions found in research literature. The basic preparation for professional practice should most certainly include the critical reading of selected studies in which research methods have been used and some "guided experience in diagnosing nursing problems, identifying rationales for implementing nursing therapy, and evaluating results in selected clinical situations."[6]

An example of exploratory study could be found in the clinic setting where the clinic nurse identifies those factors which may determine whether the patient keeps his appointment. She then selects those patients with irregular attendance and finds which of the deterrent factors were present in his clinic experience and which could be eliminated or modified by the nurse. Perhaps it was the absence of a nurse in the examining room who could protect the patient from undue exposure or who could explain procedures. Perhaps it was the lack of preparation of the patient by the nurse for the physician-patient interview or the absence of a follow-up interview with the nurse. It could be failure to explore with the patient any difficulties in transportation, home arrangements, or job requirements. Having reached some conclusions as to which factors were most often present in the clinic experience of patients who do not keep appointments, the nurse then institutes some measure to modify the clinic experience. She watches for any change in regularity with which the patient keeps his appointments.

Studies are greatly needed of factors in the home situation which affect the patient's ability to follow a medical regime or to continue a health practice which he carried out successfully in the hospital setting. What factors in the home and in the family relationships affect the mother's success in breast-feeding her infant throughout the first few months of life? Did she need help in examining the bases on which she made her decision to breast-feed the infant? Was she well aware of the requisites of successful breast-feeding? Such studies would help the nurse select not only the kind of intervention needed but when and where it should be instituted. Many failures to effect desirable change in behavior could be avoided if systematic study were accepted as an integral part of administering comprehensive nursing care.

Summary

Throughout this chapter, an attempt has been made to look at the process of evaluation to identify the requisites for evaluating nursing care. Observation, questioning, and measurement are methods and techniques which can be used in obtaining evidence of progress. Disciplined inquiry as to the results of specific nursing measures is an important part of professional nursing practice.

The quality of nursing care is a concern of many people—the patient, the family, the nurse and her co-workers, the physician, other members of the health team, and that never-to-be-forgotten aggregate called "the public." Each has his own expectations and criteria for judging what is good or desirable in nursing care. These criteria include: providing physical comfort; promptly answering requests; relieving the patient from responsibility, pain, and anxiety; assisting him in regaining independence; efficiently performing tasks; assisting in technical details; obeying orders; and acting swiftly. Nursing care can only be evaluated in terms of nursing care goals. These are established after the nurse has carefully assessed health needs and has identified those needs which can be met by nursing care. She validates her assessment by continued observation of the behavior of the patient and the family, sharing with them those nursing care objectives which she recognizes as acceptable to them. The nursing process has begun the product of which is desirable change in behavior, not only of the patient and family but of the nurse herself. Continuous inquiry and systematic listing of the outcomes of nursing action lead to sounder predictions and greater accuracy of nursing prescriptions. The involvement of those with mutual concerns in the evaluation of both product and process can result in increased comprehension of the depth and breadth of nursing.

References

1. Orlando, I. The Dynamic Nurse-Patient Relationship: Functions, Process, and Principles. New York, G.P. Putnam's Sons, 1961.
2. Bowen, E. The Biology of Human Behavior: An Integration of Sciences Applied to Nursing. New York, Appleton-Century-Crofts, 1968.
3. Fox, D. Fundamentals of Research in Nursing. New York, Appleton-Century-Crofts, 1966, Ch. 10.
4. Bloom, B.S. Taxonomy of Educational Objectives: The Classification of Educational Objectives, by a Committee of College and University Examiners. New York, Longmans Green, 1956.

5. Dumas, R.G., and Leonard, R.C. The effect of nursing on the incidence of postoperative vomiting. Nurs. Res., 12:12-15, 1963.
6. Ware, A.M. Preface to a Seminar for Graduate Students. Seattle, Washington, University of Washington, 1969.

12

Summary

The nurse must recognize the personal, inner world which affects an individual's action. She is a thinking, feeling, as well as a "doing" person. She is a product of "what has happened to her; her perceptions are what she makes of what is outside her."[1] She constantly forms new wholes within that inner world, as she sees relationships and interprets new experiences in the light of former experiences. Comprehension leads to analysis, to reorganization, and finally to synthesis. Feeling and thinking are inseparable. Response to what is happening to her becomes conscious, and values are shaped within her own inner world. The acceptance of what is good or desirable leads to a commitment to put those values into action.

A long history of emphasis upon techniques and procedures has created an image of the nurse as an action-disciplined person, one concerned with *how* an action is carried out, not necesarily *why* it was selected. Order, precision, efficiency, and, above all, command of the emotions have been the criteria most often used in planning her preparation and in judging her skill as a practitioner. In the preceding chapters, stress has been placed upon the thought and feeling behind the action. The nurse's frame of reference and what she has made of what her environment has given her will determine the completeness of the nursing process and the comprehensiveness of the nursing care given. The major concern of the nurse-educator is how to extend the nurse's comprehension to include concepts from the behavioral sciences and the humanities and to incorporate values grounded in a belief in the integrity and worth of the individual as a social being.

Any attempt to describe process is fraught with danger. "A good deal of misunderstanding among men comes from the fact they are always required by the nature of communication to make spherical things linear."[1] A process has a rhythm and cadence which escapes verbal delineation. To attempt to describe the nursing process may become an act of dissection that robs it of its vitality and its interpersonal quality. However, it is hoped that the examination of the process will bring about some reorganization in the reader's phenomenologic world, and that he will find some new meaning in the ministering of nursing care.

Administration is perceived as a part of giving as well as providing for nursing care. Wherever the patient may be—in his home, at work, at school, in the clinic, or in the hospital, and whatever his health needs may be which require the nurse's ministration, the nurse is engaged in administration as she uses material and human resources to attain established goals. She employs the classic elements of administration as she explores, proposes goals, plans, organizes, delegates responsibilities, directs, reports, and budgets time, effort, and materials. The nurse's role is one of leadership in intra- and interprofessional groups. No attempt has been made to place her in a particular setting, such as a hospital or community agency. Certainly the framework of the social setting in which she works needs to be considered carefully. This necessity was implied when reference was made to the institution's or agency's philosophy of care and to the cultural context of different professional groups. A careful study of the social setting in which the nursing process and nursing therapy takes place, has just begun. The results of such a study may resolve the conflict of the nurse-practitioner who is capable of giving comprehensive nursing care but finds herself unable to administer it in the milieu of the agency in which she works. Group experiences need to be analyzed for roles, positions and cultural patterns so that new organizational patterns may be created. These will permit the nurse to extend her sphere of comprehension and self-realization rather than to exert greater command of others.

Comprehensive nursing care requires maximum involvement of the patient and the family in identifying and assessing health needs, in setting up goals, in decision-making, in problem-solving, and in evaluating outcomes. They are truly team members and participate to the utmost of their capability. Long years of cure-directed nursing care, of doing for and to the ill patient, of instructing the well (of telling him what to do) have created a role of dependency and passivity for the recipient of nursing care and nursing services. To involve him as an *active* participant, as a learner, and as a thinking, feeling person will need careful reorientation and continued assistance in accepting a new role. He, as well as other team members, will change his frame of reference. There are evidences that this change is already beginning to take place in our society. Some measure of anxiety, discomfort, and uncertainty accompanies this change, but the patient and family will find that illness can be a very constructive experience, even though it may result in irreversible changes. He may be able to perceive health as a state of being in which he lives fully and productively with whatever resources he possesses.

The continuing effort to define professional nursing practice may become less arduous when full credence is given to the commitment of nursing to social ends, to self-realization of both the giver and the recipient of nursing care. Fortunately there is no limit to the comprehension which the individual can achieve. He always remains capable of another step forward.

References

1. Kelley, E.C., and Rasey, M.F. Education and the Nature of Man. New York, Harper and Brothers, 1952, Ch. 5.

Index